Relationships,
the Heart of Quality Care

Creating Community among Adults in Early Care Settings

Amy C. Baker
and
Lynn A. Manfredi/Petitt

National Association for the Education of Young Children
Washington, DC

Photographs copyright © by:
Hildegard Adler—166; Nancy Alexander—iv, 65, 117; Blakely Fetridge Bundy—130;
CLEO Photography—41, 48, back cover; Julie A. Correll—93; Mary S. Duru—front
cover, 68; Fotosearch—front cover; Terri Gonzalez—145; Stephanie Hynes—101;
Lynn A. Manfredi/Petitt—18, 89, 141; Paige McCray—v, 21, 160; Jonathan A.
Meyers—152; Marilyn Nolt—14, 132; BmPorter/Don Franklin—v, 28, 42, 106;
Ann Price—178; skjoldphotographs.com—97; Subjects & Predicates—iv, 35, 53, 73;
Bob Watkins—124

National Association for the Education of Young Children
1509 16th Street, NW
Washington, DC 20036-1426
202-232-8777 or 800-424-2460
www.naeyc.org

Through its publications program the National Association for the
Education of Young Children (NAEYC) provides a forum for discussion
of major issues and ideas in the early childhood field, with the hope of
provoking thought and promoting professional growth. The views
expressed or implied are not necessarily those of the Association.

Carol Copple, publications director. Bry Pollack, senior editor. Malini
Dominey, design and production. Natalie Cavanagh, editorial associate.

Library of Congress Control Number: 2004111210
ISBN: 1-928896-19-7
NAEYC Item: #156

About the Authors

Amy C. Baker and Lynn A. Manfredi/Petitt are both active national consultants, authors in the field of early care and education, and parents of grown children. Each has served as a consulting editor for NAEYC's *Young Children* journal. They are the coauthors of *Circle of Love: Relationships between Parents, Providers, and Children in Family Child Care* (Redleaf, 1998).

Amy has mentored and taught classes for urban family child care providers for more than a decade. She spent a number of years with a child care resource and referral agency and has worked extensively with the National Association for Family Child Care (NAFCC) accreditation program. She is a grant writer and a consultant for both center-based and family child care projects in Rochester, New York. She has a master's degree in English from the University of Washington in Seattle.

Lynn has worked directly with children and families in every kind of child care setting for more than three and a half decades and has served at the executive level on a number of state and national association boards. Most recently, she provides national technical assistance and shares the joys of creativity in child care centers and technical schools across Georgia. She has a master's degree in educational leadership from Bank Street Graduate School of Education.

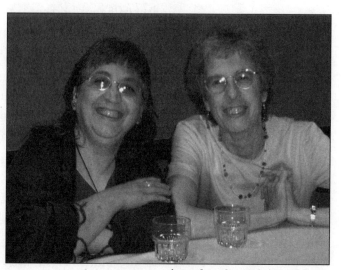

Amy (on the right) and Lynn

Contents

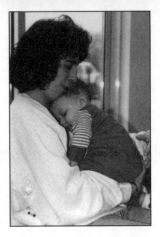

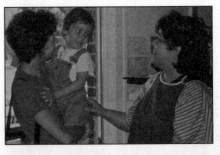

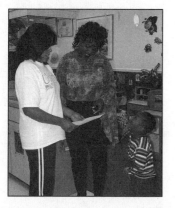

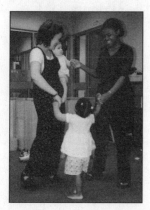

List of Boxes

Acknowledgments

We want to begin by acknowledging the two people who made this book a reality. Thanks to Carol Copple, publications editor at NAEYC, who believed in this project from the first conversation; and thanks to Bry Pollack, senior editor, who worked with persistence and dedication to bring our manuscript into finished form. We acknowledge our indebtedness to WestEd and Zero to Three for their work on caring for very young children in groups, primary caregiving, and continuity of care. We would like to thank Sid Hetzler at Splittree Farm in northwest Georgia and Stephen Luick at Allegiance Bed and Breakfast in Mount Morris, New York, where we enjoyed the beauty, joy, and incredibly large tables of their quiet writers' retreats. Nothing can beat the combination of work and relaxation that we found just a few hours from our busy daily lives. And finally, we thank each other for the enthusiasm and effort each has devoted to our long-distance partnership, which began more than a decade ago. We celebrate each other's expertise, musical talents, sense of humor, and willingness to rearrange a room—or a sentence—at the drop of a hat to make things work more smoothly.

A.B.—I want to acknowledge Elena Aguirre, director of the University of New Mexico Children's Campus for Early Care and Education, who introduced herself on a shuttle bus at a conference in Atlanta and invited me to come to Albuquerque to observe her program. Thanks too to Sheridan DeWolf and Michelle Soltero at Grossmont College, one of the demonstration sites for WestEd's Program for Infant/Toddler Caregivers (PITC), who gave so generously of their time and experience. The caregivers and families at your centers convinced me that relationship-based care isn't a pipe dream and that centers—even big ones that offer infant-toddler care—can feel like a community. Thanks too to the teachers and consultants associated with the Hanna Perkins Center in Cleveland, for the lessons you taught about the caregivers' role in children's lives. You opened my eyes to the countless ways that caregivers can support children's relationships to their parents, simply, gently, and seamlessly. Finally, I want to thank my colleagues here in Rochester. I am indebted to those of you who invited me to observe your programs (even when you knew they weren't perfect), talked openly about your challenges, and listened to what I had to say about relationship-based care for infants and toddlers. You helped me keep my feet on the ground and taught me to understand your very real obstacles. Thanks too to those of you who participate in ECDI—Rochester's Early Childhood Development Initiative. I'm awed and inspired by your dedication, vision, and willingness to collaborate. Together we're discovering what can happen when a community takes steps to work cooperatively to meet the needs of its youngest children. Finally, I acknowledge and thank my husband, Ken, for listening and giving me his loving support—no matter what.

lamp ☺—I dedicate this book to Bob Watkins, *my life partner and my heart*, and to my large, free-wheeling family (biological and otherwise!). Together you have taught me most of what I know about unconditional love. I particularly acknowledge my years at Bank Street and the focus we share on building the kind of learning communities that inspired this book. I am indebted to Bonnie Crowe and Jacob Kabb for ongoing encouragement, friendship, and dependable understanding when things got tough. My thanks go, as well, to all the Euclid/Piedmont characters—especially Michael, Wade, Louise, Jorge, and the Small family. You taught me volumes about the world of adult work outside of child care, while offering the financial stability and professional distance I needed to focus on writing. I am also grateful to the hundreds of families, caregivers, directors, early childhood students, and other professional colleagues who shared thoughts and joys and concerns about relationships—and love—with me over the years. Some of you continue to be in my life; others are delightfully rediscovered from time to time through annual Christmas cards, conference interactions, and surprise encounters at the grocery store. Even over time and distance, our bonds remain strong and vibrant. Many of our interviews were informal and seemed like casual conversation. Some of what you taught me was shared without words. I celebrate our connections and the lessons we learned together. Thanks for helping me conceptualize the wonderful things already happening in so many child care centers between parents and staff—for the benefit of the children as well as the adults. I trust that you will each see yourself in the best possible light in the words that follow. May our paths continue to cross over time.

Preface

Love is a critical ingredient in every smoothly functioning life; each one contains a caring circle of relatives and friends. Most of us form meaningful relationships naturally, surrounding ourselves with people who care about us. We work to keep connections fresh and vital. In the best of circumstances, this caring surrounds our children as well. Children thrive within webs of friendship and love. They develop their world view and expectations by living inside relationships and by observing the relationships around them. They model themselves after significant adults in their lives, with early experiences forming templates for their own relationships in later years. This happens whether the adults are aware of it or not, whether we "teach" it consciously or not. This is the way functional families and communities have been passing the gift of caring relationships along for generations.

Society in general and the early childhood profession in particular agree on the importance of surrounding young children with love. But what happens when this climate of caring is missing? What are the consequences of a child care model, serving millions of our nation's children, that does not include caring relationships as part of the deal? What happens when many of our youngest children spend most of their time among interchangeable caregivers who are business-like and distant . . . or even worse, among adults who mistrust, disrespect, or even battle one another day after day? We need to know, because that's the current climate in too many child care centers today.

Too often the center approach to adult relationships (between families and caregivers, as well as among center staff) resembles the dynamics of a dysfunctional family. All too often center policies ignore, disrespect, even disrupt, caring relationships between families, caregivers, and children. Only lately has the child care field begun to identify and address the gap between such poor practice and each child's need to be raised within a loving web of relationships. Many practitioners remain unaware of the impact it can have on the children in their care; others are aware but uncertain and confused about what to do.

To look at this issue constructively, we began to think about what we ourselves want for children. What perspectives did the two of us bring to the discussion? In addition to reading everything we could find in the literature of early care and education, psychology, brain research, and attachment, we devoured the works of spiritual writers and human potential philosophers. We were inspired by our own religious backgrounds as well as by the works of Marianne Williamson, Martin Buber, Daniel Goleman, Abraham Maslow, Pema Chödrön, Alexandra Stoddard, Thich Nhat Han, Gerald Jampolski, Paul Ferrini, Leo Buscaglia, and many others. They helped us expand our understandings of spiritual depth, human potential, and life success.

Workshops we presented on self-reflective childrearing gave us further food for thought. The many rich and honest conversations they inspired offered us insight into the values families and child care practitioners believe are important for children to internalize. We found that people everywhere want to raise children who know how to love. Love is on everyone's list. Most adults also want children to learn compassion, empathy, openness, flexibility, and a "focus on the simple, the quiet, the fun, the generous, the kind" (Rogers 1998). To that list, we added the traits of confidence, curiosity, relatedness, capacity to communicate, and cooperativeness (Zero to Three 1992). We also noted the values of the Parent Services Project, Inc. (Pope & Seiderman 2000–01), which encourages the development of joy, hope, and fun, along with cooperation, empowerment, and the ability to create community with others—critical ingredients for success at any age. During a weekend writing retreat in the mountains of northwest Georgia, we were inspired to add the importance of opening children in heart and mind to the wonder, amazement, and joy of being human and of accepting others with unconditional love. We expect this list to grow with each reader who joins our conversation.

These realizations brought us back to our original guiding principle, our shared bottom line: To thrive, children need to spend a majority of their waking hours with people who care both about them *and* about one another. The younger the child, the greater the need. Positive, caring relationships between the significant adults in children's lives are vital to quality care—no matter what the setting.

It is this belief that inspires us to share, through this book, both our concerns and the hope we found in child care centers across the country that do value and foster caring relationships between families, caregivers, and children. Join us! There's room on this journey for everyone.

◆   ◆   ◆

We are not only sustained as infants by our relationships, but throughout our lives we live and breathe relationships, whether we are aware of them or not.

—Chris Hoffman

From Our Heart to Yours

Think back to your very early years—what do you remember? Regular meals and a clean bottom? A toy-filled playroom or your napping spot? Probably not. Most likely it's the *people.* Your parents, your first tender caregivers. The neighbor who read you a book on his front step. A grandma who snuggled you close and whispered how special you were. The teacher who shared her joy of learning and naptime backrubs. The family friend who always met you with a gleam in his eye, a ready laugh, and a funny face. And wasn't your world also shaped by the interactions *between* these significant adults in your life? The respect, affection, sometimes love, they had for one another. The way they helped and supported one another.

Or maybe your earliest memories aren't so warm? Perhaps you were cared *for,* but you didn't feel cared *about.* Or instead of being part of a loving circle, you were caught in an uncomfortable tug-o-war between the grown-ups who populated your young life.

Usually a child's earliest memories are linked to people and the child's relationships to them. Everything is embedded in feelings. Everything grows out of the emotional climate and from the connections those feelings create. Experience tells us that children thrive when the adults who care for them also care about one another. When families and neighbors gather in celebration, children sense the joy of belonging to a caring community. When parents are warm and playful with each other, children feel secure and want to join in the fun; they see the world as a safe and nurturing place. On the other hand, when the grown-ups a child cares about are estranged or hostile, it's hard for that child to feel safe and to get along with anyone. Adult relationships directly and profoundly affect children's lives.

Much has been written about attachment and children's relationships with significant adults. Research on child development confirms that bonding between child and adult is critical if children are to grow into competent learners and rational adults. While bonding is the starting point of this book, our purpose is to highlight the importance of *adult* relationships in child care settings—those between parents and caregivers, caregivers and directors, and caregiver coworkers. Specifically, we explore the concept of *relationship-based child care,* the understandings and attitudes that underpin it, and the policies that encourage it. This book reflects our belief that everyone benefits when adult relationships are valued and supported alongside those between adults and children.

Finding a new model for the center setting

Over the past few decades, professionals in the field of early care and education have begun to recognize the impact of relationships in child care settings. Most of us understand that children absorb what they experience, especially in their earliest years. We acknowledge the value of warm and responsive care, and we talk increasingly about the importance of caregiver-child attachments, particularly for infants and toddlers.

We also recognize that positive relationships and compatibility among adults are good for children. Adult interactions set the tone for a classroom and, more indirectly, teach children about the world they live in and what to expect as grown-ups themselves. When significant adults in a young child's life are distant, formal, dutiful with one another—or worse, disrespectful, angry, controlling—children internalize these attitudes as characteristic of what it means to be "adult." On the other hand, when adults are warm, collaborative, and respectful, and they work at creating a caring community among themselves, children mimic that approach and carry that model into adulthood. In this way, whether or not we are aware of it, adult relationships in today's child care centers have an immediate, daily impact on children; more important, they are shaping tomorrow's adults and the future we will someday share with them.

Center policies vary considerably, even among programs with NAEYC accreditation. Some encourage family-caregiver relationships through potluck dinners, open houses, parent-initiated field trips, family bulletin boards, and weekly newsletters. Some centers urge caregivers to build and maintain adult connections by communicating

While bonding is the starting point of this book, our purpose is to highlight the importance of *adult* relationships in child care settings.

with families by phone and email, offering to baby-sit evenings or weekends, and providing other family supports. But other programs discourage parent-caregiver friendships, warning staff members to maintain "professional distance." They limit contact to short daily conversations, written notes, and formal conferences.

Sometimes a program's policies are well-meaning but short-sighted—designed to address a particular need, yet disruptive to relationships between adults. Fiscal challenge is one of the justifications most often given for practices that limit relationship-based care. The need to cover staff-child ratios and ensure safety is another. Policies that keep caregivers emotionally detached from children and their families, for example, can be the result of a program's knee-jerk reaction to those authentic needs.

Sometimes centers model their policies and expectations regarding adult relationships on what they see in the business or elementary-school setting. Child care *is* a business, but a business unlike most others. The work of caring for very young children must be viewed with a special lens, one that focuses on caring relationships that meet children's emotional needs. Everyone thrives when adult relationships in centers are more like *community* than business, more like *family* than school. In a relationship-based setting, the worlds of adults and children become interwoven. Fragmented lives are quilted into a vibrant community of strong, mutually beneficial relationships.

Early childhood professionals who resist viewing policies and practices through a relationship lens keep children from receiving the quality care they deserve. We need to take a closer look at the role adult relationships play in child care settings and the impact those relationships have on children's development. How do family-caregiver relationships affect the stability of caregiver-child attachments? How are children affected by daily tensions between parents and caregivers, among staff, between center directors and teachers? How does the caregiver-director relationship affect a caregiver's ability to offer loving care? What perceptions—accurate and otherwise—act as obstacles to centers instituting and supporting relationship-based care?

Our goal for this book is to bring a fresh focus to adult relationships in the center-based care setting. We believe it will inspire those who use a business or school model to give life to family-style relationships. We know it will give others cause to celebrate their own approach to the relationship-based model, which is being used—and used well—by high-quality family child care homes across the country and by growing numbers of enlightened child care centers. We expect this book to prompt policy makers and everyone connected to center-based settings to take the steps needed to support and strengthen caring relationships between families, center staff, and children.

Writing this book

In researching family child care settings for our book *Circle of Love* (1998), we were surprised by the number of parents who expressed the desire for a loving care relationship for their children. An overwhelming majority of high-quality family child care providers said that their relationship with children in care "feels like love." Love is a given, an integral part of the family child care program. One veteran family care provider explained, "You can't keep distance, and I don't know any day care mother who can. If you have a child for two years, it's almost like your own."

Families also told us they chose home-based care because they value a personal relationship with the caregiver. They like the informality of family child care homes, where they can talk with the caregiver at drop-off and pick-up times, sometimes even after hours. Parents said that in looking for a caregiver, they used the initial screening interview to determine whether the provider's philosophy of care and values match their own. Providers did the same, identifying families who were a good match in terms of childrearing practices and expectations. Both looked for adults who have an ability to communicate, resolve differences, and develop a strong relationship that will last for several years.

High-quality family child care offers relationship-based care. Caring parent-caregiver relationships are the norm when a small group of children and families remain in a home-based program with one or two caregivers over several years. These close adult ties benefit everyone: Caregivers feel valued and respected and free to bond with children in their care; children feel free to love their caregivers; and parents feel supported, knowing their children are happy and safe.

Knowing this, we began to wonder to what extent these benefits hold true for high-quality center-based programs. Do center staff understand the importance of relationship-based care? Do parents who choose centers hope for strong, caring relationships with caregivers for themselves and their children? Does family child care have something to teach the early care field about developing and sustaining adult relationships? For this book we examined the following questions:

- What do parent-caregiver relationships look like in accredited child care centers? Are they similar to relationships in accredited family child care settings?
- Are the caregiver-child bonds in high-quality center-based care as strong as they are in high-quality family child care homes?
- What steps have relationship-based centers taken to strengthen relationships?

In looking for answers, we observed and interviewed staff and parents in more than 50 NAEYC-accredited child care centers across the country, including private, for-profit, nonprofit, Early Head Start, and Head Start programs. We also interviewed education coordinators, freelance consultants, child care resource-and-referral staff, and educators in college settings. One of us interviewed caregivers in accredited programs in New Mexico, California, and New York. The other examined a variety of centers in Georgia and took part in countless informal conversations with students in early childhood education classes at several technical colleges. Representation among interviewees cut across geographical, ethnic, and economic lines (although many of the vignettes in this book have understandably ended up depicting some states—Georgia and New York, for example—more often than others).

Our study was qualitative and anecdotal, rather than statistical. We asked center caregivers open-ended questions about relationships with parents and children and with their center colleagues: "Do you form strong attachments to young children, or do your relationships tend to be more distant?" "How would you describe your relationship with families?" "Do you think parents understand your relationship with their children? Do they value it? How do they let you know?" "Tell me about your coworkers. How would you describe your relationships with them? Do you see one another outside of work?" "What makes— or breaks—teamwork in your center?"

We also asked directors about their interactions with families and about the director's role in the caregiver-parent relationship: "What do you do to support the caregiver-parent tie?" "How do you teach caregivers to form strong relationships with families?" "What do you do to create teamwork?" "Do caregivers have any say about whom they will work with day to day?" "What do you do to resolve conflicts?" "Are you close to your colleagues?" "How do you see yourself in relation to your staff?"

We compared the center study findings with our research into family child care settings described in *Circle of Love*. For that book we interviewed more than 75 experienced family child care providers, from all over the country, of many ethnicities and economic levels, all offering high-quality child care. Most of the providers had cared for children for at least five years, were members of family child care associations, attended regional and national family child care conferences, and were comfortable with their interactions with families.

Our understanding of relationship-based care is enriched by our extensive professional and personal experiences in child care centers and family child care homes and in the lives of family and friends. As adult educators, we have had lively conversations with practitioners in numerous workshops and college-level courses, even when relationship-based child care was not the scheduled subject. Since 1993, when we began researching this topic, we have talked with hundreds of colleagues and parents—and even the occasional stranger in the airport or on the street—about loving other people's children, caregiver-child attachments, jealousy, competition, grief and loss, empathy, communication, diversity in child-rearing styles, anger management, conflict resolution, friendship and professionalism, teen mothers, and families in crisis.

We are committed to relationship-based child care, and we are eager to share what we have learned.

1

Why Relationships Matter

Adults really count in a young child's life. The younger the child, the more important the grown-ups. We have all seen babies light up and wriggle with delight when their special people gurgle or make funny faces. A parent's look or a nod gives infants courage to crawl to the other side of the room or make eye contact with a stranger. Beloved adults have the power to soothe distressed babies when no one else can. Research only confirms what we know from experience: Children thrive when they are surrounded by people who are crazy about them (Bronfenbrenner 1991).

Life for young children is shaped by relationships. Wherever they spend their time they need to be cared for by adults who are able to invest emotionally in their well-being—adults who care *about* them, not just *for* them. Young children do best—now and later—when they are nurtured within a tightly woven web of love. A large body of research acknowledges the significance of such caring and attentive relationships. (See the range of findings in **A Look at Adult-Child Attachment** on pages 8–9.) Relationships shape a young child's growing identity (Lally 1995; Honig 2002b; Bowlby 1969): Through interactions with adults—parents and caregivers alike—infants develop a sense of who they are, what's important in the world, and how much influence they bring to relationships with other people. To develop a healthy sense of self, children need to be cared for by adults who take the time to attune to their emotions and understand their cues; long-term, stable relationships have a positive impact. It takes time and focus to get to know a child, especially one who is not yet verbal.

A Look at Adult-Child Attachment

Research on attachment supports the importance of bonded relationships between grown-ups and very young children. Here is just a sampling:

Attachment defined. Attachment is a strong emotional bond that grows between a child and an adult who is part of the child's everyday life. Attachment relationships between children and adults teach children to interpret emotions and behaviors and to develop an understanding of relationships (Bowlby 1969, 1973, 1980).

Parent-child dyad. A young child's crying, smiling, nuzzling, and lifting of arms to be carried are examples of behaviors that encourage adults to be responsive, and thereby enhance the child's chances for survival. Pediatric anthropologists note that humans have evolved to begin life as part of an intimate dyad with a loving adult. We are born before our neurology is finished; it could be said that humans really have a 21-month gestational period (9 months in utero and 12 months outside). Children are completely dependent for their survival on people who care about them. (Small 1998)

Secure attachments. Loving, trusting relationships with caring adults result in *secure attachments;* children know they can count on their adults to be attuned to their feelings and to respond quickly and constructively. Children look to trusted adults for guidance. For example, a toddler will look to his parent for a nod that indicates it's safe to explore or play with a particular toy.

- Secure attachments allow children to test the consequences of challenging behaviors—a critical part of moral and value development, or *conscience.*

- Children who have secure attachments develop resilience and a positive sense of self (Ainsworth & Bell 1974; Arend, Gove, & Sroufe 1979; Erickson, Korfmacher, & Egeland 1992). They come to believe they are lovable and important and can have an effect on other people.

- Children who have secure attachments know they can communicate their needs and will be taken seriously. These children are better at self-regulation (Shore 1997). They can comfort themselves with a blanket or a book or a teddy bear or a TV program when they need to. They're also quicker to settle down after they've been distressed (Honig 2002a, 2002b).

Attachment and conscience. Longitudinal studies show that relationships between young children and caring adults become the foundation for conscience and the capacity to succeed in school (Perry 2001). Children with poor attachment capacity are harder to teach because they feel little pleasure from teachers' warm encouraging words. They don't regret being a disappointment to adults. Conversely, children with strong attachments do better in school. They are more likely to cooperate, develop language proficiency, and have fewer behavioral problems (Perry 2001).

Attachment and emotional development. Erik Erikson's (1950) stages of emotional development create a connection between brain development and loving relationships:

- Infants develop *trust* by having physical and emotional needs met.
- Toddlers develop *autonomy* by "pushing against" loving limits of attached adults.
- Preschoolers develop *industry* through loving attention and encouragement to master skills.

Attachments with more than one adult. Children are able to become attached with more than one adult (van IJzendoorn, Sagi, & Lambermon 1992; Raikes 1993; Barnas & Cummings 1997; Goncu & Klein 2001). Children who form positive attachments to their caregivers benefit from those relationships (Honig 2002a, 2002b). Parents sometimes worry that their relationship with their child will be disturbed by a caregiver-child attachment; but relationships formed in child care don't disturb or replace the bonds between parents and child (NICHD 1991).

Attachment and brain development. The development of higher-level thinking skills depends on love and attachment. As represented in the figure below, the brain develops from the "bottom" (Bales & Campbell 2002), along the lines of Maslow's hierarchy of needs (Maslow 1970). Insecure attachments affect a child's ability to move from the brain's "emotional center," which manages trust and impulse control, to the "executive center," which is responsible for abstract thought and reasoning.

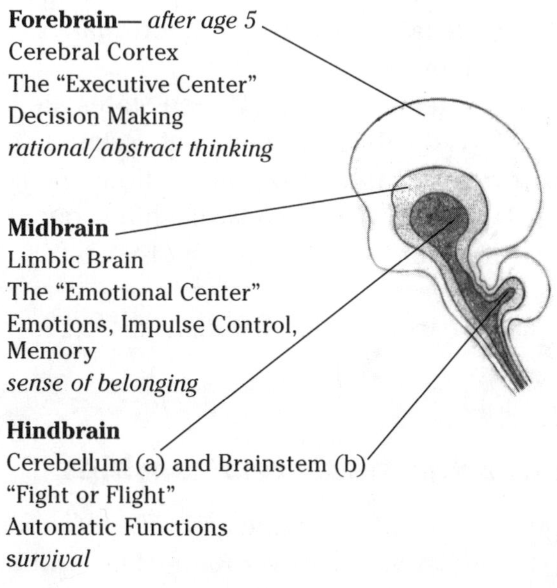

Forebrain— *after age 5*
Cerebral Cortex
The "Executive Center"
Decision Making
rational/abstract thinking

Midbrain
Limbic Brain
The "Emotional Center"
Emotions, Impulse Control, Memory
sense of belonging

Hindbrain
Cerebellum (a) and Brainstem (b)
"Fight or Flight"
Automatic Functions
survival

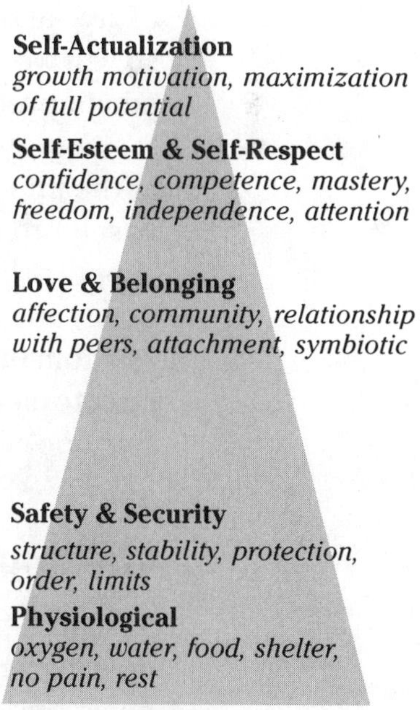

Self-Actualization
growth motivation, maximization of full potential

Self-Esteem & Self-Respect
confidence, competence, mastery, freedom, independence, attention

Love & Belonging
affection, community, relationship with peers, attachment, symbiotic

Safety & Security
structure, stability, protection, order, limits

Physiological
oxygen, water, food, shelter, no pain, rest

Maslow's Hierarchy of Needs

Children will bond with more than one adult, and that is all right. But just a few primary relationships are best when life is new. To do otherwise overloads a young child's ability to make sense of the world. Predictable adult interactions teach children what to fear, what behaviors are appropriate, how messages are received and acted upon, how to get one's needs met by others, what emotions and level of emotion can be displayed, and whether or not one is worthy of another's attention (Lally 1995). For this reason, child care should be a waltz—not a mixer dance. The field of early care and education recommends that a very young child stay with the same caregivers for the first 36 months of life, especially if the child spends more than 35 hours a week in care (Lally 1995).

To meet children's developmental needs, the daily curriculum of infants and toddlers is *relationships* (Lally 1995). But not only the relationship between caregiver and child. Relationships between adults significant in a child's life are also part of that curriculum— wherever children spend their days. In a child care setting that means parent-caregiver interactions as well as relationships between coworkers. Adult relationships have a powerful impact on children's quality of life. When adults are uncomfortable or mistrustful with one another, children feel the tension and are less able to attend to normal developmental tasks. But when adults have trusting relationships with plenty of give-and-take and care is seamless, children reap the benefits. And so will we, when this template laid down in childhood shapes their adult approach to living with others.

A growing number of centers across the United States are looking at the impact of relationships on child development. Relationship-based programs support the view that every interaction counts. We support that view too. The caregiver-child relationship is our starting point, and its development is our primary goal. But the matrix of adult relationships—parents-caregivers, caregivers-caregivers, caregivers-directors—is vital to quality care as well. That matrix is the focus of this book.

The importance of adult-adult relationships

Research has just begun to look at the nature and value of parent-caregiver relationships. The Parent-Caregiver Rating Scale, which asks questions about communication, friendship, and trust, is one example (Elicker, Noppe, & Noppe 1996). Child care professionals know that parents possess information and insights that are invaluable to their

> When adults have trusting relationships with plenty of give-and-take and care is seamless, children reap the benefits.

children's caregivers. Caring and trust enable teachers to understand a family's childrearing practices and values and offer seamless and holistic care. National standards support family-caregiver "partnerships" and encourage the professional teamwork approach to adult relationships. (See **Family-Caregiver Partnerships Indicate Quality Care.**)

Less research and practice plumbs the depths of caring relationships between families and caregivers in child care settings and the potential effects of those relationships on the children. The practice of modeling center culture after what is typical in a business or elemen-

---

Family-Caregiver Partnerships Indicate Quality Care

All national standards of excellence recognize the importance of the parent-caregiver relationship as an indicator of quality care.

National Association for Family Child Care. The NAFCC accreditation workbook emphasizes that the most important aspect of a high-quality family child care program is human interactions. The quality of a caregiver's approach to children and their families forms the foundation of support for everything else. All kinds of development are supported in the context of warm, responsive human relationships. (NAFCC 2002)

NAEYC. The National Association for the Education of Young Children accreditation criteria (1998) state that in good programs "teachers and families work closely in partnership to ensure high-quality care and education for children, and parents feel supported and welcomed as observers and contributors to the program." Revised accreditation criteria, now in preparation (2004), preserve this principle and spell out in considerable detail aspects of interactions and relationships with parents as priorities for program staff. For example, the new criteria would stress that staff need to work with families on shared caregiving issues, including routine separations, special needs, and daily-care issues.

Facilitating opportunities for families to meet together formally and informally, work together on projects to support the program, and learn from and provide support to one another is another emphasis.

Head Start. The Early Head Start and Head Start Performance Standards identify parent-caregiver relationships as a priority. Head Start involves families as partners, expecting them to share with caregivers and teachers their knowledge about their children. Parents also are asked to share in the process of planning/implementing and reviewing the effectiveness of the curriculum. (Head Start Bureau 1999)

Rating scales. The Infant and Toddler Environment Rating Scale (ITERS-R) and the Early Childhood Environment Rating Scale (ECERS), both widely used program quality scales, consider programs to be good when (1) families are made aware of philosophy and approaches practiced; (2) much sharing of child-related information occurs between parents and staff; and (3) a variety of alternatives are used to encourage family involvement. The instruments rate programs highly when families are involved in decision-making roles along with staff. (Harms, Clifford, & Cryer 1998a; Harms, Cryer, & Clifford 2003)

---

tary-school setting limits the important attachments many families and caregivers make naturally with each other. (See **The Business and School Models.**)

The Business and School Models

Business model. In the business model, service comes first; relationships are secondary. Most service-customer relationships are expected to be formal and cordial, limited to the task at hand. When we pick up dry cleaning or make a bank deposit, we don't normally tell the person behind the counter about our personal life. Mentioning visitors from out of town or a squabble with a spouse doesn't improve the service. In fact, it can slow things down. Friendships are considered messy, troublesome, and not worth the effort. Many businesses have policies against friendship with customers, among coworkers, and between staff and supervisors. Relationships are expected to be formal and limited to the work itself.

Elementary-school model. In the elementary school model, relationships generally begin and end with the academic year and are contained within the classroom. Teachers and families meet at formal conferences and have little day-to-day contact. Typically,

unless the child is doing poorly, neither parents nor teachers make a big effort to communicate separate from scheduled formal conferences. Ongoing friendships between teachers and families are not encouraged. When they do occur, they are mostly ignored unless the relationship becomes unbalanced and the teacher shows preference for one parent over others. In that case, the friendship is generally seen as unprofessional.

The teacher expects each child to fit in with the expectations of the classroom, even when there is a conflict between school and home. Little is known about the child's home life. Teachers don't usually know about changes in the family—even dramatic ones—unless the child offers the information.

The school's administrative structure supports a hierarchical relationship between the principal and the teachers. Teachers' autonomy and participation in decision-making are limited.

Likewise, little attention has been paid to relationships among caregiver team members and between caregivers and directors. We are uncomfortable with the idea of regulating emotions in the workplace— and rightly so. The line is fuzzy between what is too much closeness and not enough, between what is personal and what is professional. And yet a hands-off approach fails to take into account that such staff relationships exist, and that they can and do affect the children who also spend their days in that workplace.

Of course, not every center uses a business or elementary-school model to guide its practice regarding adult relationships. Some centers recognize that caring parent-caregiver, caregiver-caregiver, and caregiver-director relationships are the heart of quality care. Such

The Family Model

Relationship-based child care takes as its model the loving web of relationships that surrounds a child in a well-functioning extended family of parents, grandparents, aunts, uncles, cousins, and in some cases neighbors and close friends. They form a community of people who care about the child and about one another.

While no family is perfect, members of a well-functioning family try to be cooperative. They try to balance their own needs and interests with the needs and interests of others. They generally refrain from making demands that strain the ability of the rest to cooperate. Parents try to live by the rules they impose on their children; for example, if children are to resolve their differences by using words, the adults too try to settle their conflicts that way.

High-functioning families generally have a common understanding of which behaviors are permissible, forgivable, and possible—and those that are not. The adults try not to push too hard against agreed-upon boundaries, preferring community and cooperation to uninhibited self-expression. These families are resilient and flexible and able to admit new people into the circle without testing or penalties.

Members of high-functioning families generally have an appreciation of their need for one another, or *interdependency*. Broadly speaking, they have a sense of one another's strengths and know that the group functions best when everyone works together. They realize they benefit from the support and love of other family members and are able to rely on each other for help when it is needed.

Children thrive within this web of caring and usually adopt it as a template for their own adult lives as they grow.

relationship-based care, based on the family model, values and celebrates close and caring relationships between adults—whether those relationships develop naturally or require effort or encouragement to form. In such centers, relationships are as important as regulations, budgets, and the everyday tasks of caring for young children. Positive, respectful, caring interactions between all the adults in the child's world are valued as essential to the spirit, the flow, and the quality of the program. (See **The Family Model.**)

Relationship building is a priority for directors in programs following the family model. Their support and awareness maximize the likelihood of success. Valuing strong family and caregiver partnerships, directors in relationship-based programs see to it that potential caregiver teams have time to talk privately with parents who are considering enrolling their child. Directors encourage teachers to empathize with parents and appreciate the stress of raising a family while working outside the home—even if that work appears to be a choice and not a necessity. Directors also encourage understanding about the worry parents feel when they entrust their child to someone else's care. They reward teachers for going the extra mile to support families when they can, as this teacher did in one relationship-based center:

> The father realized he'd forgotten to bring his son's pacifier to the center today. He felt bad but he had to be at work and didn't have time to go home and get it. I told him not to worry. We'd figure something out. Later that morning I went out and bought the child three pacifiers to keep here at the center. I would have wanted someone to do that for me, if I was in his situation.

With a focus on balanced relationships, directors of relationship-based programs encourage parents to reciprocate caregiver kindnesses and to value the skill and commitment it takes to care for and teach other people's children. Directors help parents recognize the patience, dedication, and giftedness of the teachers and the relationships they form with children. And it works. "I don't know how my caregiver does it," says one parent, "She's so relaxed and affectionate with the children, and she almost never raises her voice. She's a gem!"

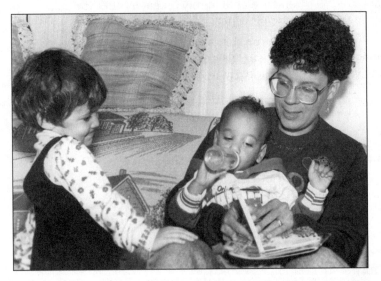

In relationship-based programs, staff interactions count too. When caregivers are hired, or need to be moved to another room, directors take into account personal styles and the relationships already formed between caregivers. Teachers who naturally get along and draw energy from each other are kept together and moved as a team. Interpersonal connections are valued, supported, and encouraged. In one infant room the caregivers describe themselves as a family and talk about what each member brings to the team:

> Sandy's the grandmother in our group. She's the one who can comfort the babies when none of the rest of us can. She just sits with them in that rocking chair and they curl up against her. . . . Denise is really good at taking pictures of the children when they are just about to learn something new. The parents love it! "Look! There's Alena discovering her toes!" . . . Ellen is the youngest member of our family and we love her. We can't wait until she's out of school and working with us full time!

Relationships, the Heart of Quality Care

Relationship-motivated directors know that caregivers thrive—along with the children—when staff relationships are full of that kind of energy and joy.

Learning from family child care

High-quality family child care can teach us a great deal about care that is relationship based. In family child care homes, relationships tend to resemble those in an extended family. Parent-caregiver connections are broad and enduring. The children in care generally get to know the provider's own children, her husband, and other family members. It isn't uncommon for a child to join the caregiver's family at the dinner table when parents are delayed. Providers often get to know the child's brothers and sisters and sometimes even go to the child's home on festive occasions.

Families and providers typically feel comfortable sharing important information about circumstances that affect the children whose care they share. Parents let caregivers know that Sam may be worried because his father is traveling or Becca might be overtired because her cousins came to visit over the weekend. Parents tell providers when household routines are changed or upset. One mother says proudly, "My caregiver knows our whole family, including our cat and dog and pet fish, and we know hers. She knows that when Grandma comes to visit, Eli is always more excited."

Parents generally say they choose home-based care because they want a close relationship with a caregiver who will bond with their child. They rely on the provider as they would an experienced family member or friend who knows about childrearing and can offer advice or help when needed. For instance, one mother who was struggling with bedtime routines asked her caregiver how she could get her child to go to bed "without three extra stories and a glass of water?" She followed the caregiver's advice and reports, "Now I have a little time to myself in the evening."

In family child care, no other adult stands between caregiver and parent; the provider is owner, director, and teacher. Families and providers sustain their relationships as long as the child is in care, and often beyond. Children who come to a family child care provider as babies often remain in care until they begin kindergarten, and many return to the caregiver's home before and after school and over school breaks. When a baby brother or sister is born, that child often follows

> "My caregiver knows our whole family, including our cat and dog and pet fish, and we know hers."

the older one's footsteps into the provider's home. The parent-caregiver-child relationship can continue for a decade or more, depending on circumstances. Friendships develop; some last a lifetime.

A high-functioning web of relationships is not exclusive to family child care. It can happen naturally and informally in any setting—and does in many high-quality child care centers. Elements of the family approach to relationships are within reach for even the largest center program. A commitment to relationships is the place to start. Inspired by the family approach, one large Atlanta center uses class trips to create intergenerational connections and community within each classroom. Children and their families, sometimes even pets, are invited to join staff and their own children on excursions. Weekend camping trips are a favorite. The adults exchange observations, casually and naturally, as they stir rice over the campfire or watch the toddlers playing. In this setting parents and caregivers find common ground and relax as peers. They bond around the children and share the joys and challenges of learning and loving.

These trips are the starting point to all sorts of adult connections within this center. The pre- and post-trip difference in relationships is dramatic. Bonds formed on these excursions are noticeably stronger than those in other centers. It is not unusual for parents who share a classroom to regularly hang out after hours with their caregiver and

---

Two Exemplary Relationship-Based Approaches

Parent Services Project (PSP). Believing that "you can't serve a child without serving the family," PSP provides training and resources to programs seeking to shift to family-centered thinking and practice. Respectful relationships are the foundation of the PSP approach, and it is built on the values of partnership, equity, shared power, social support, and asset building. In programs using PSP's approach, parents and staff work side by side to create strong and caring communities where relationships matter. All are welcome to come together to shape services and activities that meet the needs and interests of children and families at each site. For more, visit the PSP website at www.parentservices.org.

Reggio Emilia. In Italy, the community-based early childhood education approach known as Reggio Emilia creates an environment in which parents, staff at all levels, and children are involved together in continuous learning and reflection. Learning is viewed as relationship based; each child is immersed in a network of carefully cultivated, emotionally warm, and responsive relationships. Experiences of conflict and difference are valued as opportunities for discussion, repair of relationships, and reaching new points of view. The entire program culture is one of children, parents, and staff all learning and developing together. For more, see Edwards, Gandini, & Foreman (1998) and Gandini & Edwards (2001).

Relationships, the Heart of Quality Care

the children or to adjourn somewhere for supper. Community connections, once begun, endure throughout the year and even beyond; they surround the children in a circle of caring that goes beyond the norm.

The early childhood program developed in Reggio Emilia, Italy, is an example of the family approach (see, e.g., Gandini & Edwards 2001; Edwards, Gandini, & Forman 1998), with relationships one of its founding principles. Community is also an objective of child care centers involved with the Parent Services Project (PSP). Again, the sense of community and extended family is tangible among adults, with bonds that can last a lifetime. It is not unusual to discover groups of families and former caregivers enjoying each others' company at restaurants and ball games years after the formal child care arrangements have ended. Long-term relationships like these are not as rare as we once believed; they often happen naturally, even when discouraged by center policies. Slowly, thanks to programs such as PSP, authentically close adult relationships in child care settings are becoming recognized as a goal of quality care. (See **Two Exemplary Relationship-Based Approaches.**)

Benefits of positive relationships between families and caregivers

Close, caring relationships between children's families and their caregivers improve the quality of children's care in ways both direct and indirect.

Caregivers and children bond

What we learned about relationships in family child care is also true for center-based care—that a solid relationship with parents allows a caregiver to feel comfortable bonding with their child. Relationships with parents that are friendly and reciprocal make caregivers more likely to delight in children's progress, remember details to share about the day, think about the children after hours, and remain connected to the family beyond the child care years. In either setting, a child and caregiver are more likely to form strong ties when the child's parents value that relationship.

On the other hand, a tense or conflicted relationship with parents can impact a teacher's ability to become attached to their child. Many caregivers say they pull back from a child if a parent seems threatened by the affection they naturally feel for children. The warm feelings that

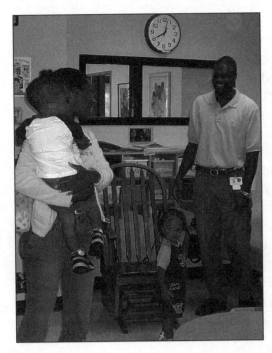

a caregiver has for children may feel uncomfortable, and even "adulterous," when parents seem jealous or insecure. Seasoned caregivers become uneasy about forming a close relationship with a child when interactions with the child's family are limited or formal. Some caregivers say they actually feel relief when a relationship-resistant family withdraws from their program, because they don't want a child whom they have grown to love to suffer an emotional tug-of-war between the adults.

Children get seamless care

Strong relationships between families and caregivers allow communication to flow naturally and smoothly. In child care this generally translates into fewer mistakes, easier adjustments, and milder upsets. Each child is better understood, and the care between home and center is seamless. An infant caregiver tells this story involving the stress of a baby's first few days in care:

> I was trying to get her to sleep, but she couldn't relax. I didn't know whether her mother rocked her to sleep or put her down and let her fall asleep on her own. I looked in her bag and found a pacifier, but it didn't seem to help. I held her on the rocker. She was exhausted, but she wouldn't fall asleep. An hour went by. I was feeling pretty frustrated because I wasn't able to help this baby, and I wasn't free to help my coworker either.
>
> After three days of this I decided I needed to talk to the mother. She told me that the baby usually went to sleep with her Pooh bear, but she didn't think we'd allow him at the center. I felt so bad! I told her we would welcome Pooh and anything else that would comfort her baby. The next day the mom brought Pooh and a beloved yellow blanket, and naptime was much easier for all of us. I rocked the child and Pooh and the blanket, and she fell asleep right away. It was such a relief!

The seamless care that results from close parent-caregiver relationships reduces confusion or tension between home and center that children may feel. A child who drinks from a bottle at home but is expected to "be a big boy" and use a cup when he's at the center will probably be confused until the adults caring for him sort out the rules. If the mother is angry with the caregiver for "making her son give up the bottle," her child will feel the tension until she and the caregiver resolve their differences.

Relationships, the Heart of Quality Care

Young children can't explain that they feel pulled in two directions. Instead they express mixed emotions through anger, aggression, withdrawal, sadness, or out-of-control behavior. In this caregiver's story, a simple connection between significant adults made all the difference in calming a little boy's anxieties and increasing his comfort within the group:

> One of my worst times was when I was caring for a little boy who came from a family who didn't speak any English. He sat in a corner for the first two weeks and cried. I tried to comfort him but I couldn't get through. Now and then I could distract him with a toy, but most of the time he sat alone. He didn't eat American food at home, and that made it even worse. I felt so sad watching that little boy. Angry too, with his mother. Why did she leave him there like that? What was she thinking? Didn't she know how miserable he was?
>
> One day the mother came to the center with a friend who spoke some English. The friend translated while I told them what was happening. I asked her to ask her son what I could do to make him happy. I was desperate. Of course he couldn't tell her. He was just 3. But he knew that his mother and I were talking about him, and that made a difference. The next day he was shy when he came in, but not tearful. He stood near the other children when they played and had a cracker at snacktime. It was because the mother and I talked that we started making progress. He didn't understand me any better than before, but he began to trust me. It took time, but gradually he became more at home in our group.

"It was because the mother and I talked that we started making progress."

When forced to compartmentalize their home and care lives, many children become overloaded. They struggle to make sense of their disjointed world but lack the capacity to make it happen. Misbehavior is a young child's way of telling everyone that the stress is too great and that the adults need to work more closely together. If the grown-ups don't compare notes, distress is inevitable for all and attachment between caregiver and child remains limited. But when adults coordinate and goodwill prevails, challenging behaviors and tension diminish and children feel as comfortable as the adults do.

Caregivers feel rewarded

The quality of the parent-teacher relationship also has a direct effect on the stability of the caregiving arrangement. Positive, caring relationships with families keep caregivers working—whether in a home or center setting. For many teachers such relationships are part of their compensation, a hidden benefit that makes them want to stick around over time (Manfredi/Petitt 1993). Caregivers are more likely to feel they are doing valuable work if they know that parents value their relationships with children as much as the mundane chores they do. An easy give-and-take with families makes teachers feel valued and validated. Reciprocity strengthens the caregiver's sense of self-worth and reduces negative feelings, stress, and burnout. This is critical in a field in which annual turnover is estimated to be 30 percent for caregivers and 40 percent for directors (Center for the Child Care Workforce 2001).

Caregivers who talk openly release conflicted emotions that contribute tremendously to burnout. Caregivers who develop a personal commitment to each family are less likely to suddenly seek other employment in the middle of a year. It is no accident that center turnover seems to be greatest at transition times, when well-loved children are moved to other rooms. Losing a group is a natural time for many caregivers to leave the job—before another group comes along to bind a dedicated teacher to yet another year of short-lived attachments.

We came across one caregiver who was well-loved by families but punished for those close ties by a new, inexperienced director. Uncomfortable with the tight, free-wheeling, confiding relationships that Val had with the "clients," the director demoted her from lead teacher. After observing this director make a particularly sarcastic remark to her, we asked Val why she stayed. Her response is a dramatic illustration of the power of family-caregiver connections:

> These are my babies! I started off with most of them in the baby room. When they moved up, I ended up taking a job in their room later that year. When they moved again, so did I. Next year they will move to preschool, and then I'll be gone—but I can't leave my babies! Besides, I know their parents so well. I babysit for some of them on the weekends, they invite me to their houses for dinner—this is my family! They know what is going on. They appreciate my staying.

Fortunately, the director of this center moved on, and the dedicated caregiver was reinstated as a lead teacher as soon as the new director learned the whole story. The caregiver still works at the center, following another group in the same way. Her kind of commitment cannot be bought. It comes from adult relationships built slowly and deeply over time.

Families return their appreciation for teacher dedication in countless ways. It can be as simple as a thank-you card or a verbal acknowledgment of how important the caregiver is in the child's life. It can be a single flower or a few tomatoes from the garden or a note written at the end of the day. In one center, caregivers in the infant room report

"I can't leave my babies! I started off with most of them in the baby room."

that parents bring in bagels or donuts in the mornings, "It makes a big difference!" Other friendly gestures, such as sharing photos of a family trip or helping pick up the room at the end of the day, are natural in budding relationships. When parents connect with them, caregivers feel less stressed by the work, and they are happier altogether. Like anyone else, when their work is appreciated and they feel part of a community of people who care about one another, even the difficult days seem manageable.

Parents relax

When relationships between families and caregivers become authentic and reciprocal, parents feel more settled and relaxed. They know they are leaving their children with people they can trust. When friction arises—and it always does—the confidence parents have in their caregivers encourages them to resolve differences rather than hide them, question themselves, or rail against their circumstances. Here's an example of a mother's confidence in her caregiver:

> I had twins and I wanted them to be fed on demand. But every time I came to pick them up, one of them would be screaming with hunger. I asked their caregiver to try to feed them before they reached a fever pitch. I hated to come to the center when one of them was crying! She had a lot of children to care for, and I knew it was hard for her to do that. I considered looking for a new center, but I liked the caregiver, and she liked me and the children, so I stuck it out. Eventually we figured it out, and my children were much happier. I wouldn't have put up with it if I hadn't liked the caregiver so much.

Once parents are comfortable, they are more likely to routinely share information about their personal interests, family relationships, and parenting issues. Family child care providers report that such information makes them better able to work through problems; it is no different in child care centers.

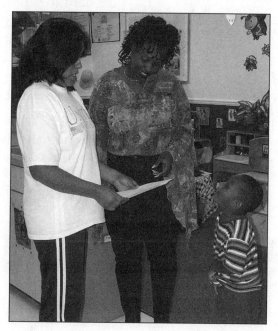

As with all good relationships, natural, informal daily interactions help everyone keep things in perspective when challenges do arise. A welcoming hello, an offer of juice or snack at the end of the day, a thank-you note, or a comfortable adult-sized chair near the doorway invites parent and caregiver to relax together and talk about the children and about their lives. The chatty bits of information easily shared at drop-off and pick-up times give the adults the insights they need to identify and untangle looming conflicts.

One caregiver tells of a child who had been taught a game by her grandfather that involved slapping him lightly in fun, then saying "sorry" and rubbing his face to make it better. When the child began playing it Monday morning with the other toddlers, the caregiver was surprised by her peculiar aggressiveness. The child was slapping her friends, but she was smiling! At pick-up time the parent's casual mention of the "Grandpa game" gave the teacher the information she needed to understand and redirect the innocent perpetrator. There was no need for a formal conference or tense telephone call. The trusting, easy interaction already developed between parent and caregiver solved the problem before it got out of hand.

Caregivers and families rely on each other

As the partnership between each parent and caregiver deepens, the inevitable differences and conflicts become part of an ongoing fabric of personal interactions rather than thorns of contention. The adults become more trusting and tolerant of each other, and solutions arise naturally and easily because of the friendship-like sharing that has formed over time. They are able to broach sensitive subjects when needed.

It's hard to separate cause and effect in good relationships. Does a teacher begin to see parents as a resource because their relationship is reciprocal and friendly? Or do families become more friendly and respectful of a caregiver because they feel valued as a resource? Either way, most of the caregivers we interviewed see families as an invaluable source of insight and information, especially when children's feelings are difficult to understand. One veteran teacher explains,

> It helps to know whether a child was up late at night when he arrives at the center tired and cranky in the morning. In the same way, it's easier to maintain a sense of humor when children throw temper tantrums if you know they are testing their parents at home too. Parents also benefit from talking to us. If parents know that their child was unable to rest at naptime, they are less likely to see him as uncooperative or "bad" when he's irritable in the evening.

Communication helps both ways, as this example offered by another caregiver shows:

> When Jen enrolled Nicky she brought a letter "written by him" about his likes, dislikes, and cues. She wanted to be sure I knew as much about him

as possible. We laughed a lot about the letter. He was only 4 months old. But it made a big difference. I knew from the very beginning I could go to Jen anytime I needed help; she made me a part of her team.

As in all relationships, the door opens most easily when time is spent mutually enjoying each other's company and sharing light-hearted conversations as well as challenging ones.

Benefits of positive relationships between caregivers

As professional organizations become clearer about their goals, they begin to set standards for themselves and their members. Our own field has a clear understanding of the importance of staff relationships.

> Developmentally appropriate practices occur within a context that supports the development of relationships between adults and children, among children, among teachers, and between teachers and families. Such a community reflects what is known about the social construction of knowledge and the importance of establishing a caring, inclusive community in which all children can develop and learn. (NAEYC 1997b, 16)

Children receive better care

Staff who enjoy respectful relationships with one another are more likely to be responsive and emotionally engaged with children in their care. Sharing the joys and challenges out loud with colleagues can help teachers to become more conscious of individual children and to remain calm, even bemused, when children misbehave or conflict. Successful caregiving teams share the workload along with the responsibility of making sure all the children are accounted for in the comings and goings of each day. Children in turn feel safe, secure, and surrounded by a sense of belonging. They are able to play, explore, learn, and cooperate with other children. The classroom becomes a happy place.

Children see positive role models

Caring, cooperative relationships between staff members model the best of adult teamwork day by day, letting it seep into each child's template for future use. Cared for by predictable adults who are flexible, responsive, and able to see children as individuals, children can afford to offer flexibility and responsiveness to others in the room. Creative exploration, humor, and playfulness take precedence over rigid rules and herd-like monitoring. When caregivers' own relation-

"I knew from the very beginning I could go to [the mother] anytime I needed help; she made me a part of her team."

ships are positive, they set a moral tone and teach children about responsibility, mutual respect, integrity, and human values in the way children learn best—through experience.

Children learn what they live, and children who live within the loving web of a bonded team are often more empathic with their peers. Here's a teacher who takes advantage of this nurturing cycle:

> A child in my care used to help other children. . . . She always looked pleased when my coworker and I would tell her that she was a good caregiver like the two of us. The other children noticed and they'd ask, "Am I a good caregiver too?" They all wanted to be like Cassie.

Families feel included

Families benefit from the stability and continuity of positive staff relationships and their children's obvious comfort in the situation. When staff members have a shared understanding of each child, parents get similar information from any caregiver they talk to. Parents feel more relaxed and confident because caregivers seem to be in accord and on top of the situation. When staff relationships are strong, families sense the respect that flows between staff members. Families feel naturally invited to become part of a caregiving team that supports one another and find mutual joy in the raising of children. Because respect and trust helps everyone feel safe, the center becomes a place where everyone can explore childrearing values and develop shared practices. Ideas and personal needs are easier to integrate when the template is already forged by bonded classroom teammates.

Caregivers feel at home

Teachers obviously benefit when their relationships with coworkers are strong and positive. They look forward to coming to work in the morning. They enjoy sharing their observations of the children. They feel understood, in accord. Their needs are anticipated. They don't have to work to assert themselves. As with good parent-caregiver relationships, staff relationships that thrive go beyond polite collegiality. Caregiver team members share their lives and values and personal challenges. Each knows what makes the others "tick" and finds ways to work around or through the difficult situations, just like a family. Here is how one teacher puts it:

> When your relationship with your coworker is good and you've worked together a long time, you don't have to wonder what the other person is

thinking. You know. You don't have to explain what you're doing either, because your partner knows. You can just concentrate on the children and do your job. The children are the center of your attention. I've worked in settings where I had to spend a lot of energy on the relationship with my coworker, and it isn't the same. When you're arguing or you have to explain a lot of things to your coworker, you can't give as much to the children. You're too busy. There isn't as much of you to go around.

The center's atmosphere is positive

People who really like and value one another pass on that positive attitude to the children. As in a fully functioning family or community, authentic staff relationships weave a safe and comfortable atmosphere where children can thrive. When staff members become comfortable, caring teams, they are actually better able to remain focused on the children in care. In settings where teachers have a strong sense of collegiality, interactions are genuine and relaxed and individuals feel free to express their thoughts openly (Bloom 1997). Conflicts resolve more easily, and each one feels supported by the others in times of stress. Friendships, often forged beyond center hours, make the center atmosphere noticeably different from less harmonious workplaces.

Teamwork is a delicate balance that must develop on its own, but that development can be encouraged. Wise administrators, Paula Jorde Bloom points out, know they cannot force a sense of esprit de corps:

> Contrived congeniality invariably backfires. A sense of community must be nurtured and developed by careful attention to the social and affiliation needs of the people who work together. [Directors] can therefore enhance collegiality by structuring opportunities that enable teachers to work collaboratively on projects, share resources, and solve problems together. (1997, 41)

Directors whose caregiving teams work well together can celebrate. One thoughtful director went so far as to *document* conversations among staff members, encouraging and valuing their interactions rather than trying to stop or control them. She created a photo essay on "collegial collaboration," which elaborated on the benefits of strong staff relationships, especially to children. Appreciative of her respect and understanding, teachers at this center use their freedom to chat wisely, constructively balancing the needs of children with their own needs for adult connections.

"I've worked in settings where I had to spend a lot of energy on the relationship with my coworker."

Benefits of positive relationships between caregivers and directors

In a traditional business or school model, power and priority are concentrated at the top and trickle down the chain of command. A relationship-based child care center functions more like a large, caring circle instead, with children at its center. Teamwork and cooperation are an expected norm for all.

Caregivers feel supported and appreciated

Outsiders may assume that because a center looks cheery, the staff naturally must get along. But positive director-caregiver relationships are not a given; they must be built over time with authenticity, reciprocity, and mutual respect. The director-caregiver relationship can be complex. The director is supervisor, mentor, check-signer, "Big Momma" or "Big Daddy," and the person to whom parents turn with complaints. The relationship a director has with each caregiver affects the way work and other relationships are approached. When relationships with the director are at their best, caregivers don't feel judged or afraid of the "boss." Instead, director and teachers operate as a professional team, pulling together cooperatively to offer the best care possible to children and families.

Caring directors are also mentors. When they enjoy mutually satisfying relationships with staff, directors become a valuable resource for second opinions and fresh perspectives about particular children or situations. The director's office can be a refuge for stressed-out caregivers or children having a really tough day who need a change of scene. Directors keep caregiver-child relationships on the high ground by being supportive, understanding, and available. Here's what one teacher has to say about her director:

> My director is amazing! I have learned so much from the way she talks to the children. She always has a smile in her voice and says just the right thing to them. I try to use her voice when I have trouble figuring out what to do with a child. Sometime it is like magic—I don't know how she does it all the time. She's like that with everybody—like a sister, friend, or my second mom!

When a staff member has a supportive and respectful relationship with the director, she can ask for help without feeling embarrassed. She may even fling herself into the director's office now and then to blow off steam, knowing she will be treated with good humor and understanding rather than disapproval. By being able to be themselves—even at their worst—caregivers are less likely to burn out. And that is good for everyone!

Appreciation from directors helps teachers see themselves as valued members of a caregiving team. Passing on compliments from parents, acknowledging progress made in difficult situations, and setting up time for teams to plan and develop their partnerships are some of the many ways that a director can show support for staff. Accommodating caregivers' personal needs, arranging for choice in professional development opportunities, and providing monetary rewards help caregivers feel valued and known by the director as individuals. Written thank-you notes and small tokens also enhance the director-caregiver relationship. In the best of centers, caregivers return their thanks to directors and coworkers, keeping the circle of community vibrant and full of potential.

> *"Some of us have been here forever—and it is all because of [our director]."*

The director-caregiver relationship affects retention (Whitebook, Howes, & Phillips 1990). With a solid relationship, a caregiver can resist the urge to take an unscheduled day off or to quit when the going gets tough. One teacher says,

> I would do anything for my director. She works harder than any of us! We can go to her with our problems—not just the ones at the center—personal things, like when I was getting divorced or when Chennee had that car accident. We are like a family. When she needs something, we are there for her too. We love her so much, we even got the mayor to declare her birthday a special day in our city a few years ago. Some of us have been here forever—and it is all because of her.

Genuine, caring relationships create loyalty that cannot be bought or taught. Director-staff interactions become a template for all other relationships in the center, establishing a foundation for quality care at its best.

Directors feel supported

Good relationships between directors and caregivers, ones that are built on respect and mutuality, are valuable to directors too. Directors need relationships to feel a part of a supportive circle of colleagues instead of a dumping ground or a buck-stopping top dog. Positive relationships with caregivers and families keep the director accessible and down-to-earth. A natural give-and-take makes the job feel doable. It's only natural if you work with people you enjoy being with, respect, and want to support that you are more likely to look forward to coming to work each day and creating a work environment that encourages everyone to do the same.

Children get better care

Respectful director-caregiver relationships offer teachers more access to information about children and their families. For example, one director changed enrollment procedures when she realized that her old method excluded the caregivers. She explains,

> I used to send a note to the caregiver with the new child's name and address. Now I'm trying harder to empower my caregivers and strengthen their relationships with the parents. I tell them more about the family when the parent enrolls the child. I might tell them the names of the child's brothers and sisters or how the parent feels about separating from the child and going back to work. If I know anything about the child's likes or fears, I pass them along so the caregiver has them from the very first day.

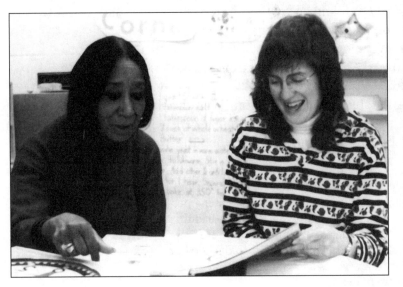

The director-caregiver relationship helps to set the tone for caregiver-parent interactions. When respect is shared, it is also passed along. In high-functioning, relationship-based centers, directors support the parents and the caregivers in equal measure. They are available to parents, but they encourage the primary relationship to be between parents and caregivers. When interpersonal challenges arise, directors bring people together and help them solve problems, rather than taking sides or being a go-between.

Including parents on the team is easy when a sense of openness and mutual support is modeled by the director and teachers. Staff with authentic relationships talk about each other in respectful and supportive terms. This allows families to feel comfortable having a relationship with teacher and director both, without the confusion of competition. Parents experience the entire staff as a team working together on behalf of the child. More voices enrich the child's experience with more input and shared expertise. Families are welcomed into the circle because the caring, respectful relationships already established between director and teachers make that circle safe, inviting, and clear.

Relationships meet our human need for community

Families, caregivers, and directors alike have told us that strong adult relationships fill a need in their lives for relationship and communal life. Relationship-based centers foster the feeling of community in dozens of small ways. Office staff are warm and friendly; they remember the names of the parents and the children and offer help even before parents think to ask. Kitchen staff smile and wave as families go by; they put out leftover snacks for parents and children in the late afternoon. Thoughtful directors show concern for teachers, and caregivers' affection for children is out in the open for everyone to see. Teachers help one another and work together with support staff as a team.

Such a center, whether large or small, feels like family. Ideally, it is a home away from home that nurtures everyone and encourages everyone to join in. Parents have opportunities to talk with other adults who care about them and their children. They get to know the parents of playmates and friends of their own children. They share a world in which the adults work together to balance work and home and meet the needs of every member, especially the needs of the very young children they all love.

◆　　　◆　　　◆

Left to our own devices, adults form positive, caring relationships naturally, especially when children are part of the mix. So why is relationship-based child care not the norm in all center programs? What challenges and dangers, both real and perceived, cause us to be cautious about, even resistant to, developing close ties within child care center culture? **Chapter 2** addresses the elements of human nature that make cordial formality between adults seem preferable to caring and connection. And it explores how centers are structured, sometimes intentionally, in ways that undermine relationship-based care.

2

When Caring Relationships Are Undermined

Our knowledge and intuition tell us to surround children with people who care deeply about them; we also know that children benefit when the adults significant in a child's life care about one another. But a look inside the field of early care and education in general and the typical child care center in particular reveals quite a bit of ambivalence, often unspoken but never far from the surface, on the topic of relationship-based care. Center administrators—sometimes unwittingly, sometimes not—establish policies that foster short-lived and unstable relationships with children and between adults. Families support those policies—sometimes naively, sometimes not—by enrolling their children in those centers and playing the roles assigned them. And caregivers enact the policies—sometimes enthusiastically, sometimes because they don't know any better, and sometimes simply because they need the job.

What beliefs lead child care centers, caregivers, and families to embrace the distance of cordial formality rather than the closeness of deeper, mutually nurturing relationships? What keeps relationship-based care from becoming the priority? People don't typically have to be prompted or forced to build caring relationships with those who share their days; they generally recognize the importance of those relationships and nurture them. To many early care professionals, doing this in a child care setting is simple and obvious. To others, it is a tall order.

This chapter examines the obstacles, both real and perceived, to creating a relationship-based focus in the center setting. The remainder of this book will look at what can—and *must*—be done to encourage caring bonds between adults to strengthen and flourish over time.

Family attitudes and feelings that undermine

Most parents know that love is key to a young child's healthy development and well-being, but they aren't always comfortable with that love coming from people who aren't kin. Their insecurities can lead them to conclude, wrongly, that their child and the caregiver shouldn't get too close and that a caring relationship between themselves and that paid caregiver is inappropriate or unnecessary.

Conflicted feelings about leaving children in care

Changing attitudes toward childrearing make it difficult for some parents to feel comfortable with the decision to put their children in care. Until a generation or so ago, a mother was expected to stay home and raise her own children, at least during their earliest years. Women who had to work outside the house usually left their children with family, kin-like friends, or neighbors—so in a sense the children remained at "home," in the community, while mother was away. Today, for a variety of economic and social reasons, *both* parents are much more likely to be in the workforce at least part time. Yet many feel ambivalent, especially about handing babies over to strangers for most of the day.

To add to their discomfort, many mothers and fathers, whether working by necessity or choice, just don't have all the time they would like to enjoy the children they parent. For many, mornings are spent rushing to get everyone up and out. Supper is picked up at the drive-through or poured from a box with milk on top. Children are fed and bathed, and everyone drops wearily into bed . . . only to repeat the routine the next day and the next. Even if parents work only 40 hours a week—and many work much more—errands, chores, and commutes occupy the balance, even on weekends, leaving little time to cuddle or play. Caregivers seem to be having all the fun.

Parents' conflicted feelings are most powerful when their children are cranky or sick. Parents want what time they have with their children to be happy. When children are out of sorts, parents don't like having to force them to get up and get dressed. They feel torn between compassion and duty when children balk at going to child care and they are late for work. They don't like being clock-watchers when children want to dawdle over breakfast. On challenging days like these, it is hard for parents to meet caregivers on even ground. Parents feel freshly judged by the world for putting their child in care and by the career choice caregivers have made to care for that child.

Some parents even begin to believe, perhaps as a coping mechanism, that their own care couldn't be as good for their children's intellectual and social growth as the care the center or preschool offers. They come to doubt their own abilities or the importance of the role they play in their children's lives. Daily time children spend away from home seems more "productive"; center staff are the professionals, the experts. One stay-at-home mother, with a master's degree in early childhood education, was confronted with that view when she was asked,

> Why isn't Leslie in school yet? Don't you know you are depriving her of important experiences? How will she cope with elementary school if all she does is stay home and play—she won't know how to adjust to different teachers! She'll think she can do anything she wants. She won't know how to work with other children. My goodness, she's almost 2! You better get busy and find a place where she can really learn!

This rebuke reflects a misunderstanding of a young child's developmental needs and the connection between attached relationships and intellectual growth. It incorrectly assumes that the roles of families and teachers are almost identical (see Furman 1986) or that out-of-home experiences are automatically superior.

Fear of being displaced

Some parents worry that caregiver-child attachments will disturb or displace the emotional bonds between them and their own children. "I was afraid my daughter believed that Nora [her caregiver] was her mommy," says one mother of a very young child. "I couldn't keep from crying. I kept thinking, I work so hard to keep us fed, and she can't even remember who I am."

Parents are the most important people in their child's life; however, child will bond to other important adults too. Research shows that additional attachments do not undermine the primary parental relationship. A longitudinal, 10-site study of 1,357 families with young children found that security of the infant-mother attachment was related to the mother's sensitivity and responsiveness. Children most likely to have an insecure infant-mother attachment were those who received the least-sensitive care from their mother and child care provider. The study concluded that "child care by itself constitutes neither a risk nor a benefit for the development of the infant-mother attachment" (NICHD 1991).

Still, parents can feel left out and jealous when a child talks about her caregiver at night or on weekends or when a child balks at going

"I was afraid my daughter believed that Nora [her caregiver] was her mommy."

home at the end of the day. One parent recalls, "I'd be glad to see him, and he wouldn't want to leave. I'd carry him to the car and he'd be crying, and I'd wonder, What is this all about? What's happening to our family? Are we doing the right thing here?"

Overprotective and competitive impulses

To care for and protect our young is part of our genetic makeup. But the impulse does not always serve the very children we care about.

> Protective urges are so strong they can lead to intense feelings and reactions in adults. When a parent places an infant in the care of a professional child care provider, the parent's natural urge to protect the child can lead to heightened emotions. Parents bringing infants to child care often have intense feelings about it, including trepidation, anxiety, and grief. They may find it difficult to trust the caregiver at first. (PITC 1997, 174)

Caregivers are human too, and they feel their own protective urges for the children in their care. Unless families and caregivers develop a good relationship, the adults may be at odds for months without ever realizing the cause of the problem.

Anytime more than one person is involved with the rearing of a child, competition between them, or *gatekeeping,* is a possibility. One thoughtful mother explained it this way to her son's caregiver, "It's not that you will make *bad* decisions for my child; it's just that you won't make *my* decisions for him." Interviewed for this book, child psychiatrist Joshua Sparrow explains that "gatekeeping," a term coined by T. Berry Brazelton, "is a result of the *passion* parents and caregivers feel for the child." (For more from Sparrow, see **Recognizing and Managing Gatekeeping** in **Chapter 3.**)

Everyone loses when adults compete for the final say or argue over who is best able to really know and nurture the child. Rather than focusing on problem solving, conversations infused with adults' passionate beliefs in their own, "right" ways, turn into a tug-o-war. Witness this one-sided complaint by a mother:

> Chaquita's teacher says that she is having trouble remembering to use the potty—but I know *my* child. She *never* forgets at home. All my other children were trained even before they were 2! Sometimes I just don't know why they hire people when they don't know the first thing about children! I told her and told her—just *remind* Chaquita and let her know it isn't okay to mess up. The teacher said she didn't think that was the "right" approach. She expects a 2-year-old to stay in diapers until she knows how to go on her own!

"It's not that you will make *bad* decisions for my child; it's just that you won't make *my* decisions for him."

Relationships, the Heart of Quality Care

For every childrearing challenge there are many appropriate approaches. Strong differences in style and opinion put children in the middle and strain relationships between families and caregivers. It is hard enough for parents in a loving marriage to sort out a shared childrearing style; with parents and caregivers it can feel like metal parts scraping against each other in an unoiled machine.

Shyness or uncertainty about sharing private information

To provide quality care requires important adults to exchange information about themselves and the children they are raising together. Changes in family dynamics affect children, so it's important for caregivers to know that Matt had a nightmare or that Mommy and Daddy are having trouble getting along, or that Grandma has come for an extended visit. Depending on the situation, a child's behavior may become more aggressive, noisy, clingy, or withdrawn. Whether or not they realize it, caregivers need parents to share personal family information in order to respond to the child in constructive ways. Conversely, parents need feedback from caregivers at pick-up time to create continuity for their child between center and home. And they all need to build the kind of mutual trust that makes this exchange possible.

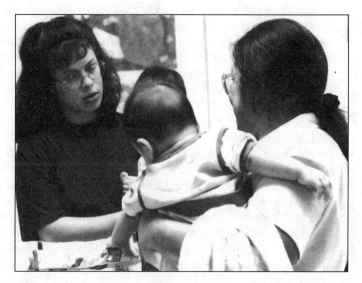

Lack of clear and complete communication leaves everyone in the dark. But how much information is too much? That's the question to consider in the story told in **Sad Little Bird** (on page 36). Like Emmal's mother, many parents who use child care are overstretched, isolated, alone, burdened; they also may be new to parenting or lack prior experience with child care. They often take their cues from center staff. If caregivers rarely ask questions or share information, parents may assume that's the norm. Some count on caregivers to know how to handle their children's behavior alone, not understanding the need for discussion about possible causes and solutions. Other parents may fear being embarrassed if they share their family's private matters or being seen as complainers if they ask caregivers for feedback.

Sad Little Bird

Emmal's mother looks around for someone to rescue her. She has been late for work three days in a row, and she's worried that this will be her last day on the job if she is late again.

"Don't worry, Emmal," Mrs. Mohar coos. "I'll be back early to pick you up."

She wishes she didn't have to leave her son so long every day. His caregiver says he is fine after she leaves, but how can she really know? What if they sit him in a corner all day? How can she be sure? "Don't cry! *Amma* [Mama] loves you. I won't be long. Oh, don't cry my little bird!"

One of the teachers approaches; she lifts the sobbing Emmal and carries him to the breakfast table, where the other toddlers are already eating. "Don't worry," Darla says over her shoulder as she plops Emmal in a chair. "He'll be fine. He's always okay after you leave."

Emmal's mother isn't sure, but she has to go. "Don't cry, my little bird. I'll be back early," she tells her son again, but Emmal still sobs. She leaves before anyone can see that she is crying too.

When Lilly arrives a little later, she asks, "What time did his mother say she would pick him up?" As one of Emmal's regular teachers, Lilly knows this will be another long day. The toddler has been coming to the center for more than a month, and he still has trouble settling down.

"She said she'd be here *early*," replies Darla, rolling her eyes. Both caregivers know that Emmal is generally the last child to arrive in the morning—disrupting breakfast—and the last one to be picked up in the afternoon.

Emmal finally calms down enough to eat some banana, but Lilly figures he'll start up all over again the next time he's hungry. Breastfed children are always like that; no one can make them happy when they want their mother. Lilly steels herself for another day of Emmal's cries: "*Amma* early! *Amma* early!"

If she could at least get Mrs. Mohar to stop saying that she'd be there early! She has to talk to her. At noon the director agrees to let Lilly make the call from her office. "But keep it short," the director says. "You know how I feel about bothering parents at work or getting too involved in their personal lives."

The conversation is short. Lilly asks Mrs. Mohar to try to get to the center before breakfast starts. She also points out that her promises of "early" don't help. Emmal just cries all day. Mrs. Mohar is stunned and doesn't say much. Lilly returns to the room feeling satisfied. She is unaware of the impact her call has had on this quiet refugee mother.

Mrs. Mohar is very upset and completely confused. Why did the other teacher tell her that very morning that Emmal was "always fine" after she left? Should she have mentioned that her car was broken down and that she and Emmal were going everywhere by bus? Should she have told Lilly that Emmal's father left them last month, or that she will lose her job if she is late just one more time? Will the center kick them out if she can't manage? And even if she could get there earlier, what can she do about Emmal's crying?

She feels lost and alone, with no place to turn.

Caregiver and director attitudes that undermine

Child care requires intimacy to navigate the emotion-laden issues that are attached to the job of childrearing. Some directors and caregivers fully embrace that intimacy; others remain wary of its implications and pitfalls. Here are some of the mistaken justifications given by programs to discourage close, caring relationships.

"Becoming attached to someone else's child is wrong"

One of the biggest challenges to relationship building between adults in child care centers stems from the cultural taboo against adults getting too close to other people's children. The taboo is one way our culture protects children from people we fear may disappear from children's lives or do them harm. Loving other people's children, especially the children of strangers, is unexplored territory for most of us, and child care professionals are the pioneers. Taboo or not, aware of the research on attachment or not, caregivers attuned to young children's needs will bond with children they care for, and most make no apology about it—"How can you care for children without loving them?" But some are nagged by worry that bonding isn't okay or professional; their fears are reinforced by some experts in the field who encourage emotional distance.

It *is* confusing. Many people aren't comfortable calling the feelings between caregivers and children *love.* We are caught off guard when caregivers are protective of someone else's child. Just how much closeness is appropriate or desirable between caregivers and the children who fill their days? Is it possible to feel too much for other people's children? Should *love* be a dirty word in child care?

"Parents don't care enough"

A good caregiver is prone to bonding and easily develops strong feelings for other people's children. This is her gift. But that same passion when misplaced can turn into feelings of competition with the parents. Sometimes a caregiver feels that working mothers and fathers have deserted their children for their own selfish goals. Such caregivers feel no sympathy when parents complain of being over-worked and exhausted at the end of the day. Some think parents put children in care because they value money and material possessions over family life. Other caregivers, believing a mother should be at home no matter what, fantasize about "saving the poor abandoned and

> "How can you care for children without loving them?"

neglected babies." Caregivers may become even more protective when a child has a bad day or seems unhappy in care; they might become accusatory, insistent, or arbitrary about changes, reinforcing parents' own anxieties and ambivalence about using child care.

Barbara is a veteran caregiver. She has worked for 15 years at a well-respected school-age child care program that is known for its long waiting list, services to children with special needs, and diverse population. Barbara recalls her initial attitude:

> I didn't know how to work with parents. I thought of them as adversaries. When they yelled at children or were rude, I thought it was because they didn't care. I didn't think they felt the way caregivers do. When they wouldn't make eye contact or were disrespectful, I thought I was more of a parent than they were. They didn't spend as much time as I did with their children. They didn't really care about their child's day.

Caregivers' negative thoughts can turn ordinary interactions with families into skirmishes and battles. A caregiver who complains to his colleague, "Angelo comes in tired because they don't see to it that he gets a good night's sleep," is setting up barriers to building a constructive partnership with that child's family.

"Caregiving and parenting aren't that different"

Some caregivers claim that the role of a loving caregiver is the same as that of a parent. Some claim to know more than the parents do about a child because "we are together eight hours a day, five days a week—most of his waking hours!" Some say it is they who are actually raising the child. In talking with caregivers, we find these misconceptions abound. Parents themselves may even feel this way at times or in some cases. When the roles are blurred, it can be confusing for both caregiver and parent—and it places stress on a child too young to understand or navigate the confusion.

In the final analysis, parenting is a lifelong role that can be shared by a caregiver for a while but never completed by her. Caregivers are knowledgeable about children in general; parents are the experts about their child in particular. Caregivers who claim to know more than the parents do about raising that child have forgotten about individual differences that only parents can know. Such claims create barriers between the adults rather than relationships.

Relationships, the Heart of Quality Care

"A 'businesslike' distance is best"

In a typical business setting we expect a certain distance between customers and the people who provide services. Beyond common pleasantries, discussion of personal lives isn't a necessity and is sometimes unprofessional. We might chat about the weather with the bank teller, but we don't expect to have to exchange personal information to get our paycheck cashed. And we certainly don't expect her to pry into our private family matters.

But the business model doesn't work so well in a child care setting. Formalities appropriate in business can act as barriers for families and caregivers trying to establish productive relationships. That's the lesson this caregiver learned:

> I called the parents "Mr." and "Mrs." for the first year because my own parents taught me that was how to address adults. When I looked around, I could see that other caregivers had better relationships with parents than I did, but I didn't know why. Once I began calling parents by their first names my relationships with them became much more relaxed.

Understandably, most people prefer not to talk about upheavals and disappointments in their private lives, especially with "strangers," and many caregivers avoid probing because it makes them feel nosy or powerless to help. But exchanging that kind of information about children's lives is necessary for quality care. When caregivers and families have only a businesslike relationship, parents feel reluctant about sharing and caregivers are hesitant about going to parents for help or understanding regarding the child. When the adults don't communicate well, small problems can become overwhelming. Children with unmet needs inevitably behave in challenging ways. Not knowing why makes it even harder for adults to understand and cope.

"Friendships are always trouble"

One reason that business discourages close personal relationships between employees and customers is the possibility of inequitable or unfair transactions if friends relax rules and bend policies for each other. The same can happen in a child care setting, if caregivers blatantly do special favors or take more time with parents who have become their friends. For families outside the circle, the inequity can be a source of hurt and resentment; they may even worry that their child is getting inferior care. Some centers take the attitude that because caregivers can't be equally friendly with every family, they shouldn't develop close relationships with any.

"Home life and center life are separate"

Most adults automatically compartmentalize the work part and home part of their lives; they are used to keeping "personal" issues out of the workplace and vice versa. But children are not developmentally able to do this; it's all one world to them. Some adults don't understand this developmental inability or they expect children to compartmentalize anyway; they resist the work required to make a child's world seamless. Teachers who view a child's home life as separate from center life don't help children maintain ties to family or to the way things are done at home. Instead, they try to redirect the child's focus to life inside the center. This attitude is most apparent when separation anxiety arises:

> If I talk about how Maliki misses her mommy, she'll cry even harder. . . . She wants to call her mother at work, but if I let her do that, she'll want to call all the time. . . . All the children will want to call their mothers! I can't let them do that!

Most of the time, a child's actions are the only way adults know something is amiss in the child's understanding of self or changing daily circumstances. When the differences between home and child care are very great, some children misbehave, others shut themselves down in one setting or the other, as they try to figure out and remember what is expected of them where—a task well beyond their capacity.

"She comes bouncing in late—in her *tennis* outfit. What does she think I am, her servant?"

Adults often miss the heart of the problem if they don't explore it together. A caregiver who tries to keep a child's life in the center separate may not initiate conversations with parents about what might be going on at home, especially if she senses serious problems. Some caregivers decide not to talk at all about it. If a child acts stressed, she might broach the child's "aggressive behavior" with the parents, but without inquiring about what circumstances might be causing it. This solution may feel more polite and respectful, and it certainly feels safer. But it leads to problems, especially if the caregiver takes sides. One caregiver learned this the hard way. She recalls, "The mother and father were fighting. The father is emotionally abusive, and so I took the mother's side. After months of this, I was shocked to discover that the father got custody of the child." Although having a close, caring relationship with both parents might not have avoided this challenge altogether, it could at least have offered the caregiver the insight she needed to help this child's mother and father redirect their focus to the child's needs.

"Can't everyone always use a hug?"

Given the needs of young children, professional child care relationships necessarily must be closer and more intimate than those in other settings. But how close? Where do we draw the line? The tendency of many child care practitioners to take care of everyone in sight—children and adults, whether they need it or not—causes some adults who are less "touchy-feely" to grimace with embarrassment. Overenthusiastic staff who are unable to adjust their emotional barometers to harmonize with more reticent colleagues and parents often cause more harm than good.

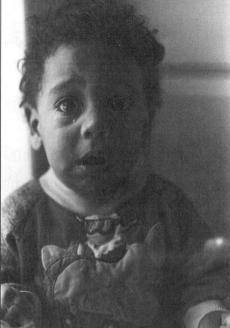

Workplace policies that undermine

Many child care programs base their relationship approach and policies on a business model. These practices have a negative impact on children by not serving their need for close relationships with just a few important adults.

"Know your place"

In the business model, employees provide services and customers or clients receive them. Maybe this hierarchical division works well elsewhere in the service sector. But when it's the policy in a child care center, an "us/them" mentality can evolve that freezes parent-staff interactions and prevents relationships from forming. Predictably, complaints begin to flow—from parents,

> She let my child get dirty and left him that way all day.

> She was all puffed up because I came to pick up my child early yesterday—it's *my* child, I can pick him up anytime I please!

and from caregivers,

> She comes bouncing in late—in her *tennis* outfit. What does she think I am, her servant? Like I have no life after work at all.

> They treat me like I am some kind of kitchen appliance that they can just plug in when they arrive and use me to cook their child all day while they are at work and not even give me a howdy-do when they pick him up.

Comments such as these indicate that close, caring adult relationships are failing to take root. Families feel disconnected from caregivers and vice versa, and each is hurt or angry about the result. Center policies that insist on "businesslike" interactions leave unspoken and unacknowledged the real need to connect, a need that goes with the territory for human beings who are trying to share the raising of children.

"Don't mix business with friendship"

In some cultures, dealings between friends and family members is normal and embraced; the trust inherent in those relationships is expected to ease the transactions. But the American business model sees personal relationships in business settings as a negative. A child care center following the business model imposes policies against fraternizing among its staff members and between staff and families because relationships are viewed as messy, unpredictable, full of unspoken expectations and subtle rules that get in the way of an efficiently run system.

Parents who are too friendly with directors might ask for leeway when they are a little short on money and can't pay tuition. They might tempt a caregiver to take their child home with her to save a late fee. They might become angry when friendship isn't enough to bend the rules, and take their children elsewhere. Staff members who become too chummy might take advantage of each other, like the caregiver who doesn't worry about arriving late because "everybody knows" that she and the director are friends. Also, failed friendships cause discomfort—even pain; and people in pain do not function well. Cordially formal interactions between adults seem safer and easier to control. While that may be true, they are barriers to forming close relationships.

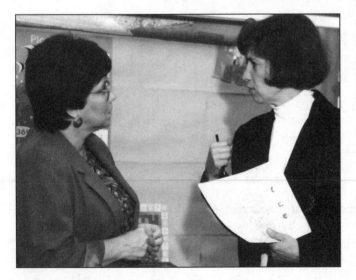

"Follow the rules . . . except when you don't"

In the business model, and even to some extent in schools, people mostly are expected to fit the system instead of the system fitting them. Certainly rules and policies are important in making an organization run smoothly. But policies that are arbitrary or rigidly enforced can be insensitive to the extenuating circumstances that arise in all our lives, especially when children are involved. Cars break down, jobs are lost, parents forget to pack diaper bags, children get sick. Sometimes people need to be cut a little slack. On the other hand, however, "slack" has a way of getting out of hand.

Too much structure puts a burden on people; too little causes the system to break down. Both extremes strain relationships between adults. For example, refusing to serve breakfast to late arrivals may keep things on schedule, but it also results in hungry, cranky children. On the other hand, stopping to serve children as they show up can be bedlam. As a balance, centers that allow a 30-minute serve-your-own-child leeway respect everyone's needs, especially the children's. Observes a director with more than a decade of experience in setting and enforcing policies:

> It can be hard to tell the hard-core manipulators from those who need a break now and then. . . . I think the key phrase is "now and then." That's why I like to have clear policies. It is easier to be aware—and kindly but *firmly* draw the line—when "one little-itty-bitty favor" here and there becomes a habit. Believe it or not, written policies make it *easier* to be friends with parents and staff.

Thoughtful policies help balance order and fairness with compassion.

"Clocks and coverage run the show"

Scheduling is complex when the needs of young children are part of the mix, especially when centers are open from 6 A.M. to 6 P.M. or even longer. Coverage requires careful juggling by the schedule maker. Full-time caregivers often get assignments between 8 A.M. and 5 P.M. or between 9 A.M. to 6 P.M. as a sign of seniority or as a perk for being lead teacher. Scheduling holes generally get filled in by floaters or part-time workers, so it's floaters who greet parents at drop-off and pick-up times and who are moved in and out of classrooms to cover staff-child ratios during absences, lunch, and breaks. In many centers, children are concentrated in fewer rooms ("telescoped") in the morning before the full staff arrives and again in the late afternoon, as the total group size waxes and wanes. This means that a child who is onsite for 9–10 hours can interact with as many as five or six adults each day—two full-time caregivers, one floater in the morning and one in the evening, and one or two floaters or administrative staff who come in while caregivers are on breaks.

Cars break down, jobs are lost, parents forget to pack diaper bags, children get sick. Some-times people need to be cut a little slack.

The younger the child, the greater the attachment need, and thus the more damaging this personnel merry-go-round can be. But defensive directors have quick answers when their scheduling decisions are questioned:

> It's only for a little bit each day. They hardly know the difference. Besides, what else can we do? It is hard to find people to work split shifts or even part time, and I can't pay someone to sit in a room with just a few children when other rooms still have a crowd!

Insensitive scheduling patterns put a strain on families and teachers as well. When floaters or part-time workers are assigned early morning and late afternoon hours, parents don't get to know the regular caregiver who spends the most time with their children during the day. If parents want to share information or ask questions, the most knowledgeable person isn't around. Or maybe, in the daily rush to get everything done, parents decide that talking with one staff member, even if he is a floater, is as good as interacting with any other. The children's regular caregiver has the same problem in reverse. Unless parents pick up children early or someone schedules a private meeting, caregiver and parents don't cross paths. Both miss the kind of information sharing that fosters good relationships and ensures seamless care.

"Follow the leader"

Another practice inspired by the business model is having the director (or other administrative staffer near the top of the hierarchy) conduct initial interviews with prospective parents. As a result, it is the director who talks with them about the services that caregivers in the level below will deliver. It is the director who questions parents about their hopes and worries regarding their children's care and shows them around the building. Rare is the director who brings new families and caregivers together to talk one-on-one.

The practice may not be accidental. It's understandable that a director would want to avoid disrupting the room by taking caregivers away from children every time prospective clients show up. And it makes sense to let families know that if problems arise a friendly expert is available. Most directors are by nature gregarious and good with people; they like to know parents and want to build "good customer relations" right from the start. If the caregiving staff changes regularly and work schedules rotate, the director may be the one character in the child care center drama whom the family sees as stable and reliable.

But some parents who establish rapport with the director never invest in a relationship with their child's actual caregiver. Given their own understanding of how business works, they see the director as the right person to come to and caregivers as less powerful and therefore less important. Teachers are left in the dark when parents speak primarily to the director, unless the director thinks to pass along the information. As a result, caregivers often feel invisible. Here's how one teacher learned that a new toddler would be joining her classroom: "The director left me a note. All it said was, 'Michael Jones will be starting on Monday,' and his birth date. I felt as though I didn't matter at all." Another caregiver complains, "When parents talk to me, they look right through me."

Many caregivers are sustained by the connections they have with families and colleagues; the relationships they form on the job are one of the benefits of working in the early care and education field. Directors who don't understand that or who undersupport caregiver-parent ties contribute to burnout and high turnover among caregivers.

Child care practices that undermine

Many centers actually have policies that discourage relationships from developing and disrupt those that do, in spite of all we know about the attachment needs of young children. Somehow the financial and personnel challenges of day-to-day center life win out over caregiving best practices. The consequences are particularly painful for children in infant-toddler care, where the developmental need is greatest for strong parent-caregiver-child ties.

Frequent moves

Many child care programs, following the elementary-school model, move children along at regular intervals. Such programs commonly move babies at 10 or 12 months, once they begin to walk, to a new room with a new set of caregivers. They are moved again six to eight months later when they become toddlers. By the time the average child in center-based care turns 3 and is ready for preschool, that child will have been cared for in four different groups by four different sets of caregivers, not counting substitutes, floaters, or new staff.

Directors and teachers in these centers cling to the belief that "life is always changing" and "children need to learn to be flexible." One director argues, "Well, that's just the way it is. . . . The parents insist that we do it this way." An infant teacher insists, "It's for the children's own safety and for their development too. Mobile infants will trip over the babies! Toddlers need more room for large-muscle activities."

Families who enter such programs find that transitions are regular and systematic, and they accept the moves as a normal and natural part of life. Some parents take comfort in their memories of elementary school and favorite teachers, reassured that a bad fit between child and caregiver will "only last a year." But they are foggy about the consequences for very young children of this "normal and natural" approach designed for children over 5. Focused on safety and ease of organization, centers fail to see the impact these shifts have on the children's emotional development. Just imagine having one new boss after another at your own job. Many of us would quit after the second or third upheaval; children in care do not have that option.

Having previously worked in a relationship-based program in New Mexico, one teacher finds the attitude at her current center incomprehensible. She struggles with the program's spoken—and unspoken—transition policies:

> The children are spending all of their time adjusting, everyone is busy grieving, and nobody is focusing on development! This is crazy. And I can't get anyone to even consider a different way. They are all wasting so much time. So much energy!

In our observations of many centers, we see children displaying a great deal of testing, tears, and disruptive behavior for as much as a month before and after each transition. Even in infant rooms, babies can sense—but not really understand—that a change is coming. When caregivers let go of their own bonds with children to deal with the change, it is confusing, sometimes even hurtful, for the children who love them.

In our experience, it takes children about 8 to 12 weeks before any transition feels complete, new relationships are established, and most seem adjusted. (Heartbreakingly, a few children never adjust emotionally to a change in caregivers.) Only then are children able to focus on other, more developmentally appropriate kinds of learning tasks. The five transitions before age 5 that are typical in center care can add up to something like a year's worth of "adjustment" during critical periods in a young child's life. Even when the transitions appear relatively smooth, children may be learning a personality pattern of easy disengagement that could be difficult to access or undo later. These annual "fresh starts" are in conflict with standards of good practice for young children.

"The children are spending all of their time adjusting, everyone is busy grieving, and nobody is focusing on development! This is crazy."

Relationships, the Heart of Quality Care

Frequent moves also take a toll on adults. Neither families nor caregivers tend to invest deeply when they know any relationship will be short term; most keep themselves fairly distant and formal—seeing this as "professional" behavior. When they know the child will be going to a new group in a few months anyway, parents don't raise concerns and caregivers don't ask parents for help. It doesn't seem worth the effort. Problems often get passed along rather than resolved. When communication is poor, parents and caregivers alike are inclined to resign themselves, make do, and hope the next arrangement will work better. Nobody wants to be accused of "making waves."

Multiple caregivers

In many rooms a team of caregivers share responsibility for the children as a group, versus pairing individual children with a particular caregiver. When responsibility is shared in this way, adult-child interactions are random. Usually the adult who is closest to a child in need responds. Often one adult focuses on the flow of activity of the group as the other adult(s) takes care of the children who are too tired or upset to keep up. For example, in infant rooms, one adult might manage the routines and the other spend time with fussy babies; in a toddler room, one teacher might lead whole-group activities while the other changes diapers and sets up for lunch. In rooms organized this way the caregivers view themselves as interchangeable, usually taking turns with chores. Children get fed, changed/pottied, wiped, and put down for naps by whichever caregiver is doing that job at the moment. It looks very efficient.

Some directors and caregivers dismiss the notion that every infant or toddler should have a special adult who cares deeply about that child. Says one caregiver,

> Children will cry or insist on only their special adult to do things for them. . . . It would be a disaster for a 2-year-old—especially for a 2-year-old! They have tantrums! . . . Children get too clingy if the adults don't change up regularly.

But having multiple caregivers—whoever is available at the moment—can make the child's world feel chaotic and unpredictable. Consider this lunchtime scene:

> Three caregivers bring twelve 1- to 2-year-olds in from outdoors, line them up to wash their hands, and sit each one down arbitrarily wherever there is an empty seat. The rules for eating are different at each table depending on the caregiver. Miss Mathews likes to talk to the children and doesn't

pay much attention to their eating habits. She permits eating with fingers, models using a spoon, and sometimes compliments the children who try to do what she does.

Mrs. Lee insists on utensils, no fingers, and punctuates lunchtime chatter with commands to "Use your spoon!" even to children at other tables. She is often observed curling a child's fingers around a spoon and guiding it firmly into his mouth.

Miss Threadgood tends to ignore the children at her table. She hops up to serve seconds to anyone who wants more. She occasionally feeds children by hand—whether they want it or not—as if they were hungry little birds. She might use a spoon and she might use her fingers. Sometimes she reaches around from behind a child without warning and pops food into an unsuspecting mouth. At her own table, children are usually left to fend for themselves while she bustles around elsewhere. They can be observed struggling with chunks of meat in unmanageable sizes, mixing applesauce and milk, smearing food on themselves, and tasting the foam plates just for fun. Their antics go unnoticed, unless someone forgets to "use your *spoon!*"

Spills and tears are routine at every table in this setting. Can't you just see Reginald playing sullenly with his spoon? Or feel the frustration of hungry 13-month-old Kendra, who is just getting the hang of feeding herself and using her fingers? Liticha needs encouragement for spoon-feeding but is ignored. Imagine the wails of 24-month-old Jamil when someone pops a lima bean into his mouth that he doesn't want. If

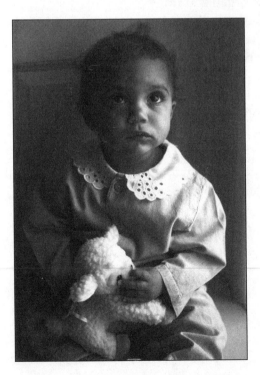

you have spent time with one toddler, you can easily imagine the frustration in this room of a dozen. It is an *un*merry-go-round that ensures daily, nonstop confusion.

When caregivers are interchangeable, children have no special person to turn to when they are tired, confused, distressed, or just needing a hug. No one is attuned to their individual personalities or temperaments. More often than not, no one spends time with them one-on-one unless they misbehave. The needs of withdrawn, shy, or quiet children can be easily overlooked. When we observed unhappy children on the playground, we asked them to tell us their teachers' names—many responded with only a blank look. They seemed confused by the very idea that they should know. Wouldn't just any adult do?

In some centers, adults are not just expected to be interchangeable; they are required to be. Some programs use smocks to designate caregivers, and keep the adults moving. This practice creates a systematic mechanism for coping with frequent changes. Children learn quickly to look for a smock; the standard name for each anonymous adult in blue is "Teacher." One center we observed even has the teachers swap classrooms daily between morning and afternoon times "to ensure coverage." Sadly, such hallmarks of institutional care are not uncommon.

Single-age groupings

In typical child care centers, children are grouped narrowly by age, usually with no more than six months in variation. The room arrangement, toys, and materials are all age specific, and special attention is given to keeping children safe. This organization has some advantages. Caregivers become specialists in the care of one age group. Those who care for 2-year-olds know what to do when children bite or throw tantrums; those with 3s know how to handle toileting accidents; those with 4s know how to deal with out-of-bounds behavior. They can tell when a child is developing typically and when he or she is outside the norm or delayed.

But in terms of relationships as well as learning, the arrangement is limited. In a room entirely of 2-year-olds, there are no older children to demonstrate the patience and self-control it takes to zip a jacket or cut with scissors. No older peers are around to serve as a model of helping those who are younger or less able; no younger children are available to inspire the practice of nurture and gentleness. Single-age groupings are devoid of the "developmental conversations" that let children know what they need to learn and where they are in relation to others on the developmental scale. Narrow age groupings also encourage comparisons between children because they focus on small developmental differences: At 11 months, Johnny might be already walking, Nita taking one step and plopping, and Vanya still crawling—is she slow? Ben is cruising and climbing and jumping; his middle name has become "No-No!"

In our observation, single-age groupings negatively impact relationships between caregivers and children. Caregivers never get to see "their" children advance to the next developmental stage. They don't get to hear beloved toddlers learn to talk in complete sentences, see them put on their own jackets, draw people and flowers, or pump a swing. One teacher laments,

> Sometimes I look at Ethan across the playground and think how big he's grown. He can run and climb up to the top of the slide. When he was in

In a room entirely of 2-year-olds, there are no older children to demonstrate the patience and self-control it takes to zip a jacket.

my room, he was just learning to walk. Sometimes I wish I could have been with him as he learned those things. We were so close when he was a baby.

The pleasure and fulfillment parents feel when they watch their own children learn and grow is denied to caregivers confined to a single-age group. A greater degree of emotional distance seems likely; so does caregiver burnout. One caregiver caught in the cycle says in exasperation,

> I just started thinking, "Won't they *ever* grow up?" and then I realized, *no!* I just keep starting over and never get to enjoy the part when they don't cry all the time or throw things on the floor or need to be changed every few hours. I get them ready for someone else to enjoy. It makes me tired.

Why should teachers invest emotionally in children or bother to get to know them well, when they know the relationship is short term?

Insensitive transitions

Transitions are always challenging. Staff often pride themselves on smoothing transition routines. Says one caregiver,

> We start children visiting their new classrooms at least a week before they are moved. Ideally we take a whole month! They make short visits at first, usually with a friend who will move too. Parents are allowed to visit with their children if they can spare the time. By the time they move, the children are ready—they start begging us to stay in their new class. When they move, they hardly miss a beat.

There is no doubt that this transition was well-planned to make changes manageable. But even well-planned transitions can affect children and the conclusions they draw from the experience about life. For example, when we questioned one child about her new classroom, she indicated that she didn't like her new teachers at all. Asked if she had told anyone, her reply was no. She said she didn't want to hurt anybody's feelings.

Sometimes only parents are aware of the toll a transition takes on their child. A mother of a rambunctious 2-year-old reveals that, although the family has moved across town, she and her husband drive the extra 30 minutes to keep their daughter in her current center:

> People think I am crazy, but I don't want to go through another upheaval like the one we had a few months ago. They had us visit a lot, and one of her teachers even moved up with the class—but her favorite teacher stayed behind.
>
> I didn't understand how close they were until Hannah began to fuss and resist after the first week and for many weeks after the transition.

"I just keep starting over and never get to enjoy the part when they don't cry all the time or throw things on the floor."

Relationships, the Heart of Quality Care

We would be heading down the hall, and she would be bubbly and happy and her old self until I turned to the left. Then she would tug on me and try to pull me to the right. If I ignored her and picked her up, she would just put her head sadly on my shoulder and say, "No, no, Mommy! No Genevieve! Miss Bethel, Miss Bethel!" (Genevieve was her new teacher in the class on the left; Miss Bethel's room was to the right.) She's finally adjusted now; sometimes they let her visit Miss Bethel in the afternoons. She seems to be enjoying life again—but that first month was terrible. I couldn't go through it again so soon.

Most parents want to cooperate with transitions, to be "good sports," and at least make it appear that their children are too. Unless caregivers and administrators communicate with families and among themselves, they may not even realize the extent of the disruption to children and families.

The risk of harm is greatest when centers move children arbitrarily and without warning, or without involving parents. Whose needs have priority when a child is moved suddenly, without peers, during a budgetary or staff coverage crisis? What happens when a center moves a child from a caregiver who loves and values him to one who doesn't? What is the long-term effect of insensitive transitions except to teach children to stay emotionally disconnected because "Life is unstable and everything changes, so it's better not to get involved."

High ratios and group sizes

We are not born in litters—and for good reason. Literally helpless at birth, human children need copious amounts of care as they undergo amazing and demanding physical, emotional, and cognitive development in their first few years. One-on-one, an adult can meet all the needs of a young infant. But even two infants is a stretch—ask any new parent of twins! Well-trained, experienced infant caregivers can do an excellent job with two or three children, but most will admit "The fewer the better!" and sigh with relief when one is absent.

In their recommendations both NAEYC (1997b, 1998) and Zero to Three (Lally et al. 1995) recognize the importance of staff-child ratios and group sizes in ensuring quality child care. For *infants,* NAEYC recommends a maximum ratio of 1:4 and group size of eight, with even lower numbers suggested as being preferable. Zero to Three recommends a ratio of 1:3 and a group size of six to nine, depending on children's mobility. For *toddlers,* NAEYC recommends a maximum ratio between 1:4 and 1:7 and a group size of 10 to 14, depending on the children's ages. Zero to Three recommends 1:4 and 12.

"I don't want to go through another up-heaval like the one we had a few months" ago.

Many states find it difficult to bring child care licensing standards in line with these recommendations. In their defense, state licensing is intended to prescribe a level that ensures *safe and reasonable* care rather than optimum growth and development. In many states the lobby for private, for-profit centers is powerful, and the desperate need for child care of any kind becomes the justification for lenient regulations. Confusing financial survival with what works best for children, many U.S. policy makers and child care professionals unfortunately have come to accept, even defend, large groups and high ratios.

The number of children each caregiver is permitted to care for varies from state to state. In New York, for example, state-mandated staff-child ratios and group sizes are close to those recommended for high-quality care. One infant caregiver in New York may be responsible for no more than four children (1:4), with a maximum group size of eight. For toddlers, the allowable staff-child ratio is 1:5 and the group size is 12. By contrast, in Georgia the allowable staff-child ratio for infants (not walking) is 1:6, with a maximum group size of 12; for 1-year-olds (if walking) it is 1:8 and 16; and for 2-year-olds the allowable ratio is 1:10 with a maximum group size of 20. Imagine changing 16 toddlers in diapers with only two pairs of hands! To their credit, many centers in Georgia keep numbers lower to deliver better-quality care; but the legal standard is mind-boggling. And in some states, the ratios and group sizes are even worse (Children's Foundation 2003).

When ratios are high and too many children are in a room, even the most qualified caregivers are unable to have the kinds of individual relationships with children and families that they know are vital. More often than not, the total group of children is managed by just one adult throughout the day, even when several caregivers share responsibility for the group. In a typical division of labor, one adult might focus on dynamics and flow, herding the entire group, while the other adult(s) focuses on chores such as changing diapers, setting up meals, cleaning the room, putting out activities, clearing cots, and so on. Under Georgia's legal standards, for example, this labor arrangement can create an *actual* ratio of one adult for as many as 12 infants or 16 toddlers. So even when ratios look okay on paper, the children's reality may be quite different.

A single caregiver responsible for a dozen or more toddlers doesn't have time to discover what makes Tim act silly, ask Carrie what she did on the weekend, or teach Denarius to make bubbles. He can't wait for Josie to think about what she wants to say about her drawing because some other child is in need on the other side of the room—crying, grabbing a toy, climbing on a shelf, or hitting a peer with a rattle. The caregiver has too many mouths to feed, too many bottoms to change, too many cots to set up to worry about individually helping each child master a new skill, laugh or sing along with him, or find comfort in his lap.

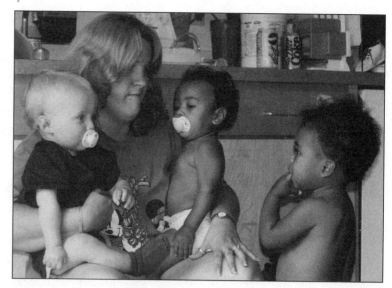

Caregivers responsible for large groups don't have time to get to know families either. Groups of 10 or more parents picking up their children pretty much at the same time means no stopping for conversation. When a caregiver has little sustained one-on-one contact with a child, what feedback could she offer that parent at pick-up time anyway? What joy or excitement of the day can she share? What can she learn from the parent to help her in her work? Even if she has good intentions, she may be so overwhelmed by the needs of the group that she gets frustrated by parents' suggestions. "They think their child is the only one in the room!"

Here's an example that clearly demonstrates the impact of ratios and group size: A few years ago a Georgia child care center was granted an Early Head Start contract that started three months sooner than expected. This forced a short-term solution of grouping four teachers and 16 children in several of the largest classrooms until the older children made their shift to preschool in the fall. This ratio of 1:4 was half the Georgia state limit for toddlers of 1:8, and it respected the state's group size maximum of 16. Outdoor play times were staggered so the children were in small groups for at least some part of every day. The arrangement seemed reasonable to administrators, but the day-to-day reality was chaos, especially during routine nurturing times such as lunch and naps. With 20 people (including adults) in one room, the noise and confusion, coupled with each teacher trying to care for all 16 children, created an exhausting environment.

Three months later the Early Head Start children were moved, as planned, to separate rooms in groups of two adults and eight toddlers each (1:4). To balance the high cost of lower ratios, tuition-paying children were kept separate from Early Head Start children, in rooms of three adults and 12 children (1:4). The quality of life improved dramatically for everyone, but there still was a difference. The rooms with 12 toddlers still felt somewhat chaotic, stressful, and herded; the Early Head Start rooms became calm, home-like models. This result is predictable: The ratios are the same, but eight children and two adults in one room can feel like a very large family, while 15 people is simply too many people living, eating, playing, and napping, all in the same room, all day long.

◆　　◆　　◆

In this chapter we examined barriers to the forming of close, caring parent-caregiver-child relationships in center settings and the effects those barriers have on the children in care. Borrowing from the experiences of hundreds of child care professionals and parents, as well as our own in both roles, we paint a picture of poor practice and rising frustration within many child care programs across the United States.

But all is not hopeless. Relationship-based child care is alive and thriving in many places. Individual centers, directors, and caregivers, as well as whole systems, are well along that exciting path of best practices. They are beckoning others to follow. The next three chapters will bring those best practices into clear view.

3

Reconsidering Individual Attitudes and Behaviors

We can overcome many of the obstacles to relationship-based care simply by re-examining and changing our personal attitudes and behaviors. Clarity in roles is key, permitting families and caregivers to relax and let relationships develop between caregivers and children as well as among the adults who share their care. Trust, respect, and sensitivity among caregivers, directors, and parents open the door to understanding and empathy, creating the conditions for a supportive and caring community to grow and thrive. Being able to distinguish between helping and interfering goes a long way, as well. Relationship-based care is new ground for some of us, but it isn't beyond our ability.

In the ideal child care world, every center would be relationship-based, encouraging (if not requiring) through its policies and practices the attitudes and behaviors necessary for caring relationships to flourish. But even without a center-wide, official focus on relationship building, individual caregivers and parents can still foster and support those connections on their own. It is possible to overcome resistance and persuade others, if we have the will to lead the way. This chapter looks at attitudes and behaviors that individual parents and caregivers can adopt to put relationship-based care within reach.

Attachment between children and caregivers is good

In relationship-based centers, directors and teachers understand that attachment is their starting point, their goal, their most important work. (See **Strategies to Encourage Caregivers to Bond with Children**

in Care.) Caregivers are comfortable bonding with young children, and directors are comfortable with these ties developing. They support one another and help parents see that a caregiver's willingness to love and to bond with other people's children is her gift—a gift that deserves to be celebrated.

Strategies to Encourage Caregivers to Bond with Children in Care

Talk in positive ways about caregiver-child attachments with caregivers, with children, and with families. Celebrate and support the growth of these bonds over time. Encourage respect for the joys and challenges of bonded children who fuss when their special adults are not around. Develop strategies for dealing with the challenges without discouraging the bonds.

Emphasize the distinctiveness of the roles of parent and caregiver. Discuss the value each one brings into the lives of children. Help caregivers understand and draw appropriate lines that balance love and professionalism in the child care center setting.

Recognize protective urges as a natural strength of both devoted caregivers *and* loving parents. Help teachers learn to understand and talk about protectiveness as a sign of their love for children. Teach problem solving and collaboration skills to diffuse adults' natural tendency toward competition for love and control over a beloved child's life.

Anticipate the grief of transitions that caregivers and children—and even parents—may feel when children must move on. To keep disruptions in relationships to a minimum: Prepare. Empathize. Involve everyone in brainstorming constructive ways for coping with and moving beyond the grief.

Adopt workplace and child care policies that strengthen caregiver-child attachments rather than disrupt them. Give everyone the security they need to believe that investing in relationships is worth the trouble. (Discussed in later chapters, such policies address scheduling, continuity, transitions, and the like.)

Attachment meets the developmental needs of young children

No matter where they spend their time—at home, with Grandma or a neighbor, with a family child care provider, or in a child care center—very young children need to be with adults who care deeply about them, and they need to bond with these important adults. Children's early relationships teach them who they are and what they can expect from the world; their healthy brain development thrives on loving attachments and a secure sense of belonging.

The best caregivers are those who are able to invest themselves emotionally and take children into their hearts. High-quality caregivers respond with compassion when children are frightened or sad. They naturally rub backs at naptime and rock babies who are too fussy to fall asleep on their own. They individualize their approaches to children, welcome their differences, and delight in their accomplishments. They open themselves to attachments, to make a difference over time even with children who come from homes where attention may be lacking. They find ways to bond with children even if other adults tell them it is "unprofessional" or "inappropriate." They instill in children a sense of being lovable, a perception that is difficult to form later in life.

The more directors and teachers value caregiver-child attachments, the better they are at speaking with conviction when they talk with families about these bonds. A veteran family child care provider prepares parents for her predictable bonding with children in this way:

> At the very first interview I tell parents I will fall in love with their babies and their babies will fall in love with me. If parents are unhappy with that, they don't choose my care. They may decide to stay home with the child . . . or they may go to another provider or to a center. But this is the way it is at my house. This is how it has to be—children need to be with people who love them.

In the typical center setting, caregivers are not usually present during first interviews with parents, but sensitive directors set expectations for parents similar to those set by this family provider. When parents need help sharing their children and letting them bond with caregivers, strategies such as the ones in **Helping Families Value Caregiver-Child Attachments** (on page 58) offer a good place for directors and teachers to start. Not all parents find it easy to acknowledge the importance of attachment. Some initially feel threatened by the idea of love shared between their child and the caregiver. The good news is that this understanding is teachable, and within reach. Families sometimes need help to understand why a caregiver would be delighted at a child's arrival or to appreciate her sweet, snuggly kisses at pick-up time. Many parents need reassurance when they see the caregiver and their child exchanging hugs, or when the caregiver jumps up to attend to their child even when they—the child's own parents!—are present.

Parents often have to be taught that a caregiver who loves other people's children—who regularly beckons, invites children to her lap, and keeps them close for bottles or stories—is a person to be cherished and treasured. Love is not diminished when it is shared. Understanding that idea helps parents value the child-caregiver bond right from the start. They can see that children are happiest when they are

Helping Families Value Caregiver-Child Attachments

Talk about attachment and relationships at the initial interview or as soon as a family enters care.

Help parents understand children's need to form attachments—especially infants and toddlers—with the special adults who care for them, regardless of the setting. Explain that a young child is able to bond with multiple significant adults, but that just a few is best.

Celebrate the primary attachment between parents and their children. Caution parents against behaviors that destabilize that connection, such as sneaking out without saying good-bye.

Talk about children's happiness, how they thrive when they are with people they love who love them back. Connect this to brain development and identity formation. Show how attachment to caregivers frees children to focus on more developmentally appropriate tasks of childhood and builds the foundation they need for higher-level thinking as they approach age 5.

Explain that high-quality caregivers are distinguished by their ability to bond with other people's children. But also share what professional lines your center has drawn to keep its approach to caregiving respectful of family bonds, appropriate, and constructive.

Describe what your center does to acknowledge and support children's attachments to beloved caregivers. Go over program policies that keep center attachments intact over time in order to give bonds a chance to be effective. Explore strategies to cope with children's grief at losing those bonds when they must move on.

with people they can openly love and who openly love them back. As one enlightened mother explains,

> I wanted someone I could be friends with and someone who would love my child. I've been very happy with Joan. She loves Stacy, and Stacy loves her. When I see them hug each other I know I've found the right person for my child. That bond is exactly what I was looking for.

Parents like that one also deserve to be cherished and treasured.

Children can love more than one adult

Research and experience both show us that child care by itself constitutes neither a risk nor a benefit to the mother-child attachment. Longitudinal studies on the impact of child care on family relationships show that the babies who are the most likely to have *insecure* attachments to their mothers are those who have received the least-sensitive care from their mothers and their child care providers (NICHD 1991). Children who are deeply attached to their mothers still can become attached to other special adults who care about them (Howes 1999). Loving, daily contact forms a strong, lasting bond between a child and parent. Some parents still worry that caregiver-child attachments will disturb their parental bond, and they fear that their child's attachment to them will be damaged by so many hours of separation. Sharing the concepts outlined in **Sharing the Love** can help to comfort parents who remain wary of child-caregiver attachment.

Gatekeeping is evidence of attachment

Competition between adults over who has the final say or who is *best* able to nurture a child is a possibility whenever care of that child is shared. That parents and caregivers have differing views on childrearing also can bring out protective urges that trigger such "gatekeeping" (Brazelton 1992; Brazelton & Sparrow 2002).

Gatekeeping, as understood by T. Berry Brazelton and the staff of the Brazelton Touchpoints Center, is a sign that strong bonds are forming with the child, and although it can be stressful, it is also a good sign. One solution to the tension is for parents and caregiver to *stop,* and recognize the caring in each other's approach—that is, the wish to offer the best possible care to a child who is so well loved. See **Recognizing and Managing Gatekeeping** (on page 60) for more suggestions for developing adult relationships in the child care setting.

Sharing the Love

Parents and caregivers will be more comfortable with relationship-based care and strong child-caregiver attachments if they can be helped to understand these things:

Children can love many people—mothers and fathers as well as grandparents, aunts, uncles, cousins, special neighbors, church members, and other adults whom they get to know over time. A child comes to love a good caregiver in the same way. Attachments are often the result of time spent together.

There is enough love to go around. Just as children are able to love both parents at the same time, the parent connection is not diminished if children love their caregivers too.

The child-parent relationship cannot be duplicated. It will last a lifetime. Caregiver-child attachments may be strong, but they are limited by duration and intensity.

Permission for relationships to develop comes from parents. They choose the care setting; they keep the family's connection to a caregiver alive over time—or not—once the caregiving arrangement is over.

Relationship-based care helps children maintain family ties while family members are apart. Centers with a relationship-focused approach actively and consciously support the child's home life and love, even while he enjoys life and love at the center.

Recognizing and Managing Gatekeeping

Gatekeeping urges are biologically driven responses of adults to attachment behaviors of newborns and young children, speculates child psychiatrist Joshua Sparrow, director of special initiatives at the Brazelton Touchpoints Center and an assistant professor at Harvard Medical School. This biological factor explains the intensity of the response, says Sparrow, in an interview for this book. "Caregivers and parents both want to do well for the child, but it ends up as competition for who is *best* able to nurture (or know) the child. Often it is up to the caregiver to guide parents through their insecurities and grief to a place of openness and mutual support."

The Center promotes a positive understanding of the gatekeeping phenomenon in its work with care professionals. Addressing the potential for gatekeeping in advance—before it comes up—is the most constructive approach. "No fault—no blame. Celebrate it as a norm that identifies the real caring of adults," encourages Sparrow. He offers these additional suggestions:

• Help parents value and recognize that child care professionals are profoundly undervalued and in a challenging job. Support one another and understand the toll it takes to "fall in love with children in care, knowing that you must give them up at the end of each day."

• Help parents appreciate caregivers by making small everyday gestures—notes, smiles, food—and by sharing themselves in open, authentic ways.

• Value and validate the contributions parents and caregivers each make to the child's life. Look at what is positive in the child's development and notice out loud how each adult has helped bring it into being.

• Understand each adult's vulnerability in feeling strongly bonded with the child. Parents and caregivers both are in mourning for having to greet and lose a well-loved child day after day. Support each other in this grief that the two roles carry.

• Use the Touchpoints principle of using the child to develop deepening levels of relationship with parents:

Level 1: Compliment the child in generic ways.

"What a beautiful baby! Look at those eyes!"

Level 2: Make positive, specific observations about the child's behavior.

"I can see that she is a friendly child." "Look how he smiles at me."

Level 3: Make observations about the child's behavior that can be attributed to the parents' parenting abilities. Gift the child's parents with a validation of their unique connection to their own child.

"See how she waited until we spoke a while before she let me hold her. She wanted your approval before leaping into the unknown with a stranger. That shows she is very attached to you. Look how she works to keep you engaged!"

• Remember and promote the belief that all parents are the experts on their own children and want to do the best by them. In the same way, remember and promote the belief that all caregivers are experts on children in general and want to be competent with all children in care.

About Touchpoints. The Brazelton Touchpoints Center (BTC), based at Boston's Children's Hospital, offers training based on the work of Dr. T. Berry Brazelton. The training combines relationship building and child development into a framework that care professionals can use to enhance their work with families.

Contact. Website: www.Touchpoints.org. Email: Touchpoints@tch.harvard.edu. Phone: 617–355–2297. Related books: Brazelton (1992) and Brazelton & Sparrow (2002).

Parenting and caregiving are different roles

A clear understanding by adults of their particular roles in a child's life helps them welcome the child's relationships with multiple loved ones. Secure in this understanding, the parent is able to give to the child permission to reach out to others. No bond competes with the one she has with Mommy or Daddy—not even the ones she develops with teachers Lynnie and Louie at the child care center.

What caregivers do is not parenting

A caregiver is paid to act as a parental substitute, hired to act on the parents' behalf in their absence. While a caregiver does many of the things that parents do when they are with their children, she doesn't replace them. The misconception that a parent's and a teacher's care for a child are no different may grow out of the notion that child care is a matter of tasks rather than of relationships (Manfredi/Petitt 1993).

How do caregivers learn to see their role as different from that of a parent? How do they discover their limits? An experienced toddler teacher gives us a clue:

> I used to think I was doing as much as the parents were. I was with their children so many hours—sometimes 10 hours a day. The consultant at our center helped me sort out the differences in our roles. Parents have a commitment to their children that will last for their whole lives. They're responsible when their children are preschoolers and when they go to elementary school and high school and when they learn to drive and when they go to college, if they do. Sometimes parents are even responsible for their children after they become adults. Our commitment as caregivers is short term. We have the children for a year or two in the daytime. We don't have them when they're sick or at night, and we get time off on the weekends. . . . Another difference is that we are always with children in groups. Most parents have one-on-one time—even if it's in the car on the way home. We rarely have just one child all to ourselves.

The box **The Role of Caregiver vs. Parent** (on page 62) expands on these differences. We can also look to the children themselves for information on how the roles of parent and caregiver differ. As Dombro and Bryan note in their book *Sharing the Caring* (1991), children tend to trust their parents more than they trust any favorite caregiver. They save their biggest hugs *and* their most emphatic no's for their parents.

Families are relieved when they see that the caregiver's role is collaborative and complementary rather than competing. Remember the mother in **Chapter 2** who complained, "It's not that you will make

"Parents have a commitment to their children that will last for their whole lives."

The Role of Caregiver vs. Parent

There are a number of distinctions between the role of the caregiver and that of the parent. Here are some of the most important contrasts.

Caregiver's role in a child's life	Parents' role in their child's life
Relationship is short term.	Relationship lasts a lifetime.
Relationship develops mainly during child care hours; responsibilities do not extend beyond.	Bonding begins at birth, some might say even earlier; responsibilities extend 24 hours a day for many years.
Child seldom has caregiver's exclusive attention.	Child often has one-on-one time with parents, and shares them only with siblings.
Caregiver is *an* important person in the child's life.	Parents are *the* most important people in their child's life.
Caregiver tends to be objective about the child's behavior.	Parents tend to be emotional and biased about their child's behavior.
Caregiver is unlikely to know the child's extended family members, neighbors, or friends. Child usually does not know the caregiver's family or communities.	Parents are the hub of their child's nuclear family. They link the child to the extended family and various communities.
Caregiver is trained in and expected to use professional early childhood guidelines more than cultural, social, or personal preferences in her interactions with the child.	Parents are not usually trained in child development; they usually follow cultural, social, and personal preferences in raising their child.

bad decisions for my child; it's just that you won't make *my* decisions for him"? With her developing relationship with the caregiver, the mother gained a new insight:

> After months of exchanging values and child-rearing opinions, my caregiver and I had come to know each other so well that she *was* making my decisions—and I was making hers. I realized that we had developed a reservoir of shared understandings. I was able to trust Anna in ways I hadn't believed possible when we first met.

This trust became the foundation of a close relationship between parent and teacher that lasted throughout that caregiving year. When they accidentally bumped into each other five years later, the pleasure they felt at reconnecting was that of old friends.

It isn't always only the parents who are relieved, as this teacher explains:

> Once I began looking at my job this way [as complementary with parents] it became less stressful, knowing that my relationship to the children has limits. I love them, but they aren't my complete responsibility.

An administrator of a child care program in California echoes this point:

> Our caregivers are facilitators. They support the child's independence, and they encourage the child to value his parents. When caregivers understand their role in this way, they feel relieved because they know their role in the child's life is limited. They can comfort children, rock them, hug them, sing to them, and even love them, but they can't do what their mothers or fathers do. And that's all right.

Supporting the parental bond is part of good caregiving

Relationship-savvy caregivers don't try to usurp the parental role, but instead help children maintain relationships with their parents in a setting that meets the children's developmental needs. We saw this wisdom put into practice in a child care center in Cleveland, where the caregiver, Carla, supervised toddlers in a large classroom. As parents said good-bye, she positioned low stools at the window overlooking the parking lot so the toddlers could see their parents leave for work. After a few minutes of watching, one of the children began to cry. "You got those missing-Mommy feelings?" Carla asked matter-of-factly. "You want to sit on my lap for a while?" The little boy rubbed the tears from his eyes and shook his head no. Carla didn't ask again. Instead, she invited him to join a group of children working on a project at one of the tables, giving him an alternate way to cope with the pain of separation. In another toddler room, the caregiver, Angie, helped a child with her coat. "Is this how your mommy does it?" she asked. The child nodded. Later when one of the children was in wonder over a beetle, Angie said encouragingly, "We'll tell your mommy you were wondering about that."

These two teachers don't expect a child to forget his parents, Grandma, or Poppy upon entering the center. *Mommy* and *Daddy* aren't words to be avoided in their classrooms. Neither is *love*. Good teachers remember and evoke children's thoughts of the parents in their absence. Family habits and traditions are valued as guides for caregiving and as touchstones for a developing child. Caregivers understand their role is to act on parents' behalf, doing the mommy and daddy job until pick-up time.

A family child care provider named Laura told us she prefers to care for children who have at least one adult at home who "loves them fiercely," or as attachment expert Alice Honig likes to say in addressing caregivers, at least "one person who acts like the sun rises and sets on their child." Without fully understanding her own motives, Laura guided one mother into a deeper bond with her challenging toddler, but let another child go because his parents were too detached. She tries to bond with the children in her care without creating loyalty conflicts or confusion. Because she knows that a child's most important bond will always be with that parent, relative, or guardian at home, she is always looking for ways to close the gap between home and child care. Teachers who understand their caregiving role this way can actually help parents realize their importance to their children (Furman 1987).

Some caregivers learn to value and celebrate the parent-child bond by working in settings that make clear what children's relationships are to their families. Here's how one teacher learned:

> We had a consultant in our center who kept telling us that we had to do more to support the child's feelings for his mother because it was his most important relationship. I had trouble with that, especially with mothers who didn't do things the way I did. . . . [For example] I had one family who slept with their 3-year-old in a family bed. I didn't like it because I thought children that age should be more independent and sleep on their own. When the child was cranky or overtired I'd think, "It's the parents' fault; the child doesn't get enough sleep." The consultant said I should try to think about it from the parents' point of view. Why do they sleep with the child? What are they thinking about? She told me if I couldn't figure it out on my own, I should ask them. I decided to ask—as neutrally as possible. They were very straightforward. They said they never had enough time with her during the day because they worked so many hours, and this was one way they could feel like a family at night. It was warm and cozy in the morning, and they had a few more minutes together when they woke up. After that conversation I began to look at parents differently. Knowing they had reasons for doing what they do made it easier to support them.

"**Knowing [the parents] had reasons for doing what they do made it easier to support them.**"

Another caregiver, in a middle-class urban neighborhood, came to the same conclusion by a different route:

> When I first heard I had to support family relationships, I felt put upon. I felt like it was asking for too much. The first time I told a child, "I bet your mommy will be interested in knowing you were thinking that," I felt like I was in a play, reading a script. But the words made a difference. The child remembered and told his mother, and she became more friendly and approachable. As our relationship changed, I began to feel that she was supporting *me*. Supporting a child's relationship to his parents makes good sense now. We need to support one another.

Relationships, the Heart of Quality Care

A young child cannot compartmentalize

When we remember how the brain develops (as discussed in **Chapter 1**) and look at the emotional development of young children, it is easy to understand why seamless care is so important. Identity formation takes place in the earliest years. Significant aspects of the way that adults act are perceived, interpreted, and incorporated into the child's developing sense of self (Lally 1995). Adults' actions teach children how to behave, what is expected, how other people should be treated, and how children should feel about what is happening to them and around them (Lally 1995). The closer significant adults are to one another in values, style of living, and expectations, the easier it is for a young child to incorporate these aspects into a clear sense of self.

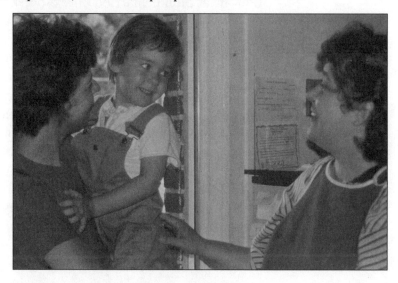

Because they cannot compartmentalize their world as adults can (into "work" and "home," for example), children find gaps and discrepancies between settings and particular adults confusing. Like a computer with too much data to process, the younger the child and the larger the gap, the more time and energy it will take the child to make sense of the chaos and establish the developing self.

Center and home both leave their mark

Generally, a child's deepest, long-lived relationships are established within the family during the first few months. Foundations for growth are created; the family style of nurturing, communicating, sharing, and so on, forms a blueprint for that child's life. Family relationships are touchstones for a child's sense of how things are (and should be) done and what is important. The same thing happens to very young children in child care. Their child care relationships also are touchstones, imprinted in this same way. Infants carry the memory of the way they were held or tended to by their mother (or primary "mothering" person); they imprint her way of responding to them, the way she talked or tickled or sang to them. As toddlers, interactions with their special, loving adults teach children self-control, negotiation, pride, shame, and the way it feels to share positive emotions.

Young children carry these early imprints wherever they go and into whatever they do. In a humorous example, consider the aware and very verbal 3-year-old who asked how it was possible that a certain couple she knew could be married. Careful questioning revealed the source of her confusion: All other couples in her life happened to share the same color hair, but this couple didn't. Fortunately her misconception—that blonds married only blonds, and so on—was harmless. But not all of life's imprints are so innocuous. Tracing the roots of such imprints and undoing their consequences is even more challenging when the important adults in a young child's life are not discussing values or exchanging details of daily life.

Developmentally unable to compartmentalize, young children merge their child care setting into an extension of what they think of as "home." One 3-year-old, during a comfortable transition from a toddler classroom of eight children to a preschool classroom of 20, proudly announced, "I used to live in a little house, but now I live in a *big, big* house!" He was telling us something about how he views his world. He doesn't separate his life in the same way that we adults do. He uses the word *house* to describe the place where he lives with his classmates and teachers; it is the same word we use to describe the place where he lives with his parents and siblings.

Children shouldn't have to choose

Because children cannot compartmentalize, the web of adult relationships in child care (among family members, between parents and caregivers, among center staff) should resemble a well-functioning extended family. In other words, for optimum results, children's developmental work is best accomplished in a *holistic* world, a seamless world of support created by important adults working closely together on the child's behalf. Children thrive when all the important adults in their lives share similar values, have compatible expectations, and develop routines that are more or less consistent. Children are confused when their experiences in one context clash with their experiences in another, especially if the contrast is great. Young children are not developmentally ready for this kind of variation on a theme. The caregivers and families who help children thrive are those who keep the differences—especially those between center and home—simple, clear, and easy for children to manage and understand.

When adults' actions and expectations do clash, the child feels confused and emotionally torn. Under such conditions, even something minor can spark behavioral challenges.

> Three-year-old Rachel is new to the center, and at naptime she confidently begins pulling off her shoes and socks. She can't understand why the caregiver is telling her to leave her shoes on. Shoes aren't allowed on the bed at home, and her mother praises her when she takes them off on her own. Rachel is too young to understand why her caregiver wants her to sleep in her shoes—what is a "fire drill" anyway? Conflicted, but most comfortable with her mother's rules, she is determined to take her shoes off. Naptime at the center becomes a daily power struggle. Rachel protests and cries and tries to take off her shoes. The caregivers, who push her shoes back onto her feet each day, get progressively upset at her stubbornness. Finally, in an emergency phone call conference, Rachel's lead caregiver and her mother realize that the rules at the center differ from those at home.
>
> Only by making this discovery are the adults able to help Rachel deal with the differences between these two worlds that she sees as one. Once Rachel realizes her mother and her caregiver are in agreement, she is able to relax and happily follow the solution they work out: to wear her shoes at naptime for the "short sleep," but remove her shoes at home at nighttime for the "long sleep."

"Once Rachel realizes her mother and her caregiver are in agreement, she is able to relax."

Tension can result when significant adults in a child's life have incompatible expectations, even when they are as minor as shoes on or off. Children's unease increases if adult relationships are strained or if important issues are at stake. Here's an example reported by a program in Cleveland associated with the Hanna Perkins Center:

> Teachers were frustrated with the new little girl in their classroom, who cried a lot and refused to take part in activities with other children. They were reluctant to approach the child's father because they had come to view him as a "frightening, bad guy." Most of the time, they avoided him and tried to handle things on their own. They suspected the 4-year-old was reacting to parental discord at home, but they were hesitant about talking to her about her feelings. On the one hand, they worried she wouldn't tell them anything, which would bring them right back to the father; on the other, they were afraid she'd reveal something shocking. With help from a consultant, the teachers realized they might be the cause of the tension. By letting the girl see them avoiding her father, the teachers were unconsciously asking her to choose between him and them—to compartmentalize her home life and her center life, which she was incapable of doing. So they began to talk constructively with the father and to say positive things about him to his daughter, and soon the child became more relaxed and cooperative. Relieving her of her dilemma made all the difference. (adapted from Streeter & Barrett 1999, 169)

Knowing each other personally is good

Mutual trust and understanding between parents and caregivers help caregivers manage those trying days when children are restless, cranky, whiny, or simply unhappy. Trust and understanding enable all the adults to work through or let go before misunderstandings get out of control. When parents and caregivers understand and care about each other, caregivers are able to remind themselves that a parent having a bad day is greater than the sum of his or her behaviors, and parents can remind themselves that caregivers can be trusted to have good intentions. Their positive relationship makes the adults feel safe in asking each other for help when tempers flare.

Warm, trusting relationships develop from the little things, such as casual chitchat at drop-off and pick-up times. Caregivers who value relationships take the lead with parents, sharing stories about the child's day and remembering to ask (without being intrusive) about things going on at home ("How was Jamie's visit with Grandma?"). Parents offer family information, and ask caregivers for insight or advice about child care ("Angel is having nightmares about turtles— any idea why that might be?"). As the adults become more comfortable with each other, they begin talking about themselves, maybe about what's going on in the office, what they did last weekend, or even where to find a good mechanic.

By talking naturally this way, parents and caregivers do more than share information: They give each other glimpses into their personal

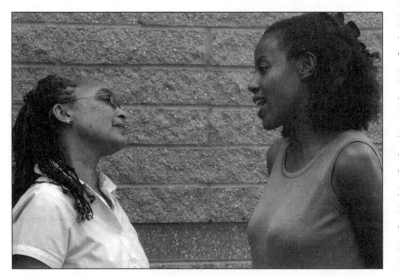

lives. With time and established rapport, each conversation builds on previous ones. The adults come to really know, understand, and care about each other. Everyone benefits—caregivers feel supported, parents feel cared about, and children are able to observe and enjoy the bond growing between their most important adults. Some parents and caregivers may even form genuine personal friendships.

"Professionalism" means integrity, not distance

Early childhood centers that value relationship-based care understand "friendship" and "professionalism" in new ways, and they follow a model that fosters caring connections between adults. They accept close bonding between adults as normal—even as *likely* in a setting populated by the kind of person who readily comes to love and care for other people's children. And they anticipate that some parents and caregivers will become closer than others.

Close relationships and actual friendships can even be a goal, as long as they do not interfere with the needs of other children and families in the center. Inside the child care setting, no parents should be made to feel that they (or their children) are less important to a caregiver than her friend is. The center's director and teachers must remain balanced in their judgments of the various families and take a conscious, thoughtful approach to managing adult relationships. NAEYC (1997a, 1997b) recognizes the importance of this balance when it defines *professional* relationships between caregivers and parents as "partnerships" and advocates ethical standards, such as avoiding preferential treatment and protecting confidentiality.

It is when centers or caregivers equate "professionalism" with keeping emotional distance that problems for children arise. Although child care certainly is a business, children are not served by centers that follow the business model of employee-customer relations, in which staff are expected to be "professional" by being impersonal, emotionally disengaged, punctual, orderly, and the like. Following the business model in a child care setting means devaluing attachment and limiting the natural inclination of caregivers to connect and empathize with children and families. Instead, relationship-focused programs promote the family model, teaching professional integrity and encouraging close relationships and friendships. Caregivers feel supported; their natural abilities to bond and intuit emotional needs are enhanced. Caregivers and parents rearing children together are free to follow their instincts and treat each other in ways that help everyone thrive.

To get the benefits of relationship-based care, we must draw new lines between openness and privacy, friendship and formality. For many, this requires a new kind of thinking about parent-caregiver interactions and the boundaries set in the typical center-based setting. The director of a small NAEYC-accredited center talks about how her

> To get the benefits of relationship-based care, we must draw new lines between openness and privacy, friendship and formality.

As staff members . . .

• examine current practices that impact adult interactions and decide on ways to make relationships blossom. For example, does the daily schedule allow regular caregivers to meet parents at drop-off and pick-up times?

• talk about professionalism. What does it mean to be professional? Is it possible to have a personal friendship as well as a professional relationship with a family?

• discuss "friendship" and the center's policies (formal or assumed) about adult relationships.

• develop written policies if none exist. If possible, include parents in the process.

• discuss current matches between families and caregivers. Are the pairings working? Are any mismatches? Every relationship is different, of course; but the really problematic ones stick out. Should some classroom assignments be changed?

• learn problem-solving techniques and conflict-resolution skills to work through issues that prevent both friendship and professionalism from thriving.

With families . . .

• plan relaxing, playful events that encourage comfortable interactions and authentic relationships to develop and grow between caregivers and families—for example, a swimming party, a family-staff field trip to the circus or a basketball game, regular potluck supper nights.

• explain and discuss policies that staff have developed to encourage a sense of community and connection and enhance relationship-based care.

---

perceptions of what really counts in quality child care were changed by a gifted caregiver who knew that what counts is *relationships*:

> Our 3-year-old classroom had a lot of turnover this year. We only had one caregiver who stayed throughout the year, and I had lots of reservations about her. She was good with the children, but she wasn't good with paperwork. Her room was always messy, and her relationships with the parents were way too noisy and excitable for my taste. I felt as though I'd let the families in that room down, that we hadn't given the children much in the way of quality care.
>
> At the end of the school year this caregiver decided to take a different job. The parents held a good-bye picnic for her. Every parent came, and that doesn't happen very often. When the caregiver arrived—she was a little late—the children and parents flocked around her. They laughed and wished her well, and the children gave her presents. They all had a wonderful time. Several of the parents took me aside and told me what a wonderful year it had been for their child. They *loved* Miss Rose.

The box **Drawing New Professional Lines for Adult Relationships** offers strategies to help staff negotiate new relationship boundaries. When staff explore this boundary concept together, they also learn self-reflection and team-building skills. Staff members who construct their own knowledge about professional limits are more likely to use those boundaries appropriately and be able to articulate them both to parents and to new staff members. This builds a program culture that is predictable, stable, and full of professional integrity.

Connecting is contagious

Many individual practitioners are already talking about balancing warm, adult relationships and professionalism. A part-time caregiver assigned as a floater in a large program recalls how her chance connection with a parent had an effect on everyone's relationships and attitudes:

> Taylor was a young 3 when he started at the center, and I noticed that he was unusually fearful. (I didn't know it until later, but Taylor had been a premature baby and had some brain damage.) I always thought of myself as fairly likeable and easy to get along with, but this child would sit in a corner far away from me anytime I was running group time. He was somewhat comfortable with the regular teacher, but I saw him shy away from her too, and I knew she saw him as a troublemaker. He was too clingy

---

How Directors Can Foster Parent-Caregiver Bonds

Celebrate and call attention to adult relationships that make things work more constructively for the children (between director and caregivers, among caregivers, but especially between caregivers and parents).

Teach caregivers empathy and communication skills. Talk with them about their attitudes toward families. Encourage them to look for parents' strengths, not their shortcomings. Emphasize that parents love their children and are doing the best they can.

Build empathy in parents toward caregivers. Talk with them about their attitudes toward caregivers. Encourage them to look for caregivers' strengths.

Mentor caregivers and parents in forming relationships with each other. Model relationship building for caregivers and families alike.

Hire caregivers who display relationship-oriented dispositions—that is, who can accept differences in childrearing, who express empathy for working parents.

Orient new caregivers and new families to the importance of building relationships with each other.

Arrange opportunities for caregivers and families to interact informally. For example, encourage informal conversations at drop-off and pick-up times.

Create safe places where caregivers can vent frustration and deal with challenges away from parents. Teach conflict-resolution skills; make sure the skills are used and reinforced.

Adopt workplace and child care policies that foster the formation of close adult relationships rather than disrupt them. (Discussed in later chapters, these policies address scheduling, continuity, transitions, and the like.)

---

and afraid and took up too much of her attention. I never saw any of the full-time teachers hug or cuddle him or go out of her way to establish a relationship with his mother. They always said, "He needs to learn to get along" or "His mother really spoils him!"

One day I met Taylor's mother in front of the building, and we started up a conversation. She told me how much he loved my group time circles. I was floored! He apparently knew all the songs we sang, and sang them to her at home. She and I talked about music, and while we were talking, Taylor was a different child. With great delight, he started running back and forth between us and the door. Each time he came back, he hugged his mom and laughed. As she and I became more and more comfortable with each other, he began to hug me too, every other time. His mother expressed surprise. She said he had never hugged any of his teachers before. I think he felt safe with me because he could see that his mother and I made a connection. Her body language and smiles made it okay.

Taylor and I were always comfortable together after that. This family has shown me how much of a difference my relationship to parents can make to the children. When we adults are distant, I think children mimic that distance. If we become relaxed and friendly, it changes everything. Actually, the change in Taylor toward me seemed to make the other teachers look at him and his mother differently too.

Instead of waiting for chance encounters, relationship-based centers take steps to help connections happen. **How Directors Can Foster Parent-Caregiver Bonds** (on page 71) offers some tips.

Empathy comes from understanding

As adults come to know each other, they become more emotionally generous, relaxed, and empathetic. Empathy is an important feature of relationship-based care. Empathy allows parents to feel understood and welcome; it helps caregivers feel connected to families. Chances are the adults also will be more compassionate when children are irritable or teary or overtired, because casual conversations help everyone understand the reasons for the behavior. Empathy is the key in the following story of a caregiver who developed a warm, supportive relationship with a mother living in a homeless shelter.

I had an 18-month-old named Alton who wouldn't lie down on his mat or fall asleep. He'd cry and carry on and disturb all the children. The other teachers thought he was spoiled. The boy's mother was very young. She had a know-it-all attitude, and she would sort of go deaf whenever we tried to talk with her about Alton. Most of the staff decided it was her fault that he was so hard to settle at nap, and [they] resented both of them for making their days so difficult. . . .

Late one afternoon the mother and I got to talking. I told her about my daughter and shared some of my concerns as a parent. She told me

"[This child] and his mom taught me a lot of things. I learned that I don't hold anything against a kid once I get to know the mom."

Relationships, the Heart of Quality Care

that before she became homeless she used to be a nanny and that the child's mother taught her a lot about raising children. I asked, Did Alton ever nap? Yes, she said. But because [in the shelter] there wasn't a clean place to put him down, he always slept on her chest. I knew this shelter. It was filthy and a little bit scary. This mom was shy and quiet compared with the other residents. Most of the women fought with each other, and it wasn't uncommon for them to beat their children. She told me that the other mothers made fun of her for being too protective. They thought she should spank Alton or at least put him down. . . .

I began to think that the mother put on an "attitude" because she wanted to protect her ideas about childrearing. She didn't want the rougher mothers to know her soft side or get her to stop doing what she believed was best for Alton. That realization made it easier for me to feel compassionate toward her child. I tried lying down with this little boy on my chest, and it worked. He fell asleep in 30 seconds! It was easy as pie to roll him gently onto his mat—and he stayed asleep. . . .

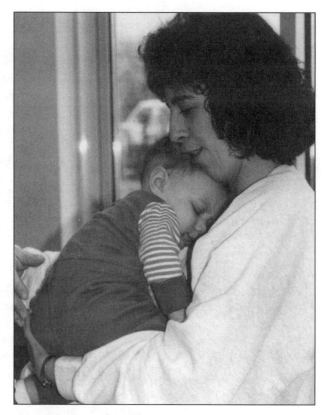

He and his mom taught me a lot of things. I learned that I don't hold anything against a kid once I get to know the mom. A child doesn't feel like a problem once they are both a part of my heart.

It isn't always easy to empathize with someone who does things differently from the way we would. It's even harder not to be judgmental when children we have come to love are involved. Just listen to some veteran caregivers talking about their childrearing values, their frustrations, and the differences they have observed over the years.

Children just aren't being raised the way they used to be.

One of the changes I see is that parents are less willing to discipline. We've seen 5-year-olds still in cribs because the parents can contain the child there, and they can't do it any other way.

Children don't know how to relax and put themselves to sleep the way they used to. At home they watch TV and fall asleep. Or they sleep with their parents. Or the mother gets up once they're asleep and carries them to their rooms. When we started caring for children, out of a preschool class of 16 children, 14 would nap. Now only three sleep.

How We Think Affects Our Ability to Empathize

Attitudes/beliefs that prevent us from feeling empathy	Attitudes/beliefs that allow us to be more empathetic
Talking about the feeling will only make it get stronger. *"She seems to miss her mother so much . . . so I avoid mentioning the topic."*	Talking about the feeling may make it grow stronger at first. But then it may lessen because someone understands and cares. *". . . so when I mentioned her mother, she started crying. I hugged her until she was ready to get down and play."*
We want the feeling to go away. *"That mother seems angry . . . so I just ignore her."*	Once it is acknowledged, the feeling will weaken, maybe even disappear. *". . . so I said I felt the same way sometimes, and we began to talk about it. Really talk. Now we get along great."*
We want the person to be more positive. *"We all have problems . . . he just needs to get over it."*	The person's ability to cope may strengthen once the difficulties are acknowledged. *". . . so I told him it had happened to me with my own child, and we began to compare notes."*

Clearly some children don't eat dinner at the table. We can tell because they fall out of their chairs. They don't use utensils.

They come when they have colds and they'd rather be home in their PJs. They come when they have fevers. Parents take the child's temperature and then, three hours later when the fever is down, they send the child to child care. . . . Children don't get vacations, but parents do. We're the ones who have to deal with children's feelings about this during the day. We tell parents, "Stay home with your child some days when you are on vacation."

Of course, caregivers aren't the only ones with frustrations. Parents' empathy skills are challenged too, by caregivers who refuse to use pacifiers, insist that children arrive "on time," or make little ones walk instead of being carried. But differences are less likely to become complaints when caregiver and parent have the kind of close, authentic relationship that allows each to see the situation from the other's perspective. For more, see **How We Think Affects Our Ability to Empathize.**

There are many "right" ways to rear a child

It is no simple challenge for people to rear children together, especially when they find that their childrearing values and practices differ. Childrearing differences can exist between spouses, between parents and grandparents, as well as between families and caregivers. Cultural, social, and economic background is a big factor in shaping a person's thinking about the "right" way to rear children. But even among people with similar backgrounds or who live in similar circumstances, individual approaches to childrearing can be very different.

Many adults—even some early care and education professionals—assume that "everyone" rears children the way they do (or everyone *should*), until they are shocked to discover that "everyone" doesn't. Some can articulate their childrearing values (Mrs. Lee's "Use your *spoon!*" for example), others may not have thought them through so consciously. Differences that exist between parents and caregiver, for example, may not be apparent initially. Often differences do not reveal themselves until they cause a problem or become the focus of a gatekeeping conflict—unless someone knows to ask about values in advance.

Navigating differences constructively is critical

Recognizing that there are many good ways to rear children is one of the entry points to relationship-based care. Appreciating this truth enables us to be more respectful, understanding, and even curious about other adults' interactions with their children. It can be freeing to realize that some of us feed babies on demand, and some of us try to keep to a schedule. Some parents expect their child to finger-feed himself as soon as he is able; others feed their child with a spoon until she can eat without making a mess. Some caregivers expect preschoolers to dress themselves; others believe it's the adult's job. Some mothers encourage children to play in the sandbox; others don't like dirt or grit. Some fathers talk to newborns; some don't or think it's silly. Some parents use candy to motivate their children; others never give their children sweets. One mother at a local book club shocked some of her neighbors—and was applauded by others—when she announced proudly: "Harmony is 4 years old and she has never wiped her own butt—and I am not sure she *ever* will! I'm not going to keep rinsing out nasty underwear when I can keep it from happening by wiping her myself."

"It helped
that I didn't
insist that
they do at
home what I
do here. And
it helped that
I believed in
what I was
doing. Neither
way is really
wrong."

It's easier to manage the differences when we allow for a variety of possibilities. Once their significant adults are clear and in sync about expectations, it's easier for children to manage the differences as well. The caregiver who doesn't cultivate this critical professional perspective usually burns out in frustration, leaving the sharing of childrearing to those more tolerant, easy-going, experienced, and flexible. Or they find themselves locked in conflicts with parents over whose way is "best" for the child. Veteran caregivers often develop strategies in advance—or by default—and take the lead in helping everyone find a place of comfort when conflicts rock deeply held beliefs.

One teacher explains that when there are big differences between home and center, she consults the family and tries to "explain as reasonably as possible what I do and why I do it. This approach has got me by with parents—even when we agree to disagree." She recalls a mother and father who were shocked to hear their son calling genitals by their anatomical names.

> I told them that's how we do it here. Not [every family] uses the same nicknames, but anatomical names are always the same. Besides, a child needs to know the terms that doctors and other people use. I told them that if they wanted to use nicknames at home, that was all right with me. . . . That worked for them. It helped that I didn't insist that they do at home what I do here. And it helped that I believed in what I was doing. Neither way is really wrong.

A similar approach works for another caregiver who is particularly bothered by preschoolers who are used to eating from their parents' plates:

> These children aren't given plates or bowls of their own. They're fed on their parents' laps. It might be all right to do this at home, but when they come to day care and sit at a table with other children, it's a big problem because they take food from their neighbor's plates. I can't blame them. They weren't taught differently. But the other children don't like it. I have to separate them and teach them to eat their own portions. . . . At first, I didn't know how to talk with the parents about this. I didn't want them to feel I was judging them. I talked about it with my director, and we decided to tell them that for health reasons we don't let children share food or drinks. Diseases pass quickly when children are together, and we have to take precautions that parents might not have to take at home. This worked pretty well. The parents didn't feel judged, because they knew the situation is different in day care.

Expertise in child development helps negotiate some childrearing differences. Here, an experienced caregiver used her knowledge of children's needs to explain her philosophy of care:

The grandfather of a Chinese child wanted staff to follow his lead and carry the child most of the day. He diapered his granddaughter on his lap and anticipated her needs before she could express them. I couldn't do that with a group of babies, but I didn't want to tell him that. And I wanted him to let her follow the American pattern. . . . So I explained that I wanted the child to learn to calm herself and to express herself in words, and told him it would help her later on as a bicultural citizen. . . . It took several weeks of his watching, but eventually he was able to trust that I was taking good care of his child—in the American way.

Often the best strategy is to find a way to laugh about the issue, or to let it go as quickly as possible. Knowing when to press a point and when not to is one of the secrets to developing good relationships with parents. It is a skill worth perfecting, as this caregiver has:

Sari was only 10 months old and her parents were already spending every spare moment doing educational and enrichment activities. I thought about trying to get them to slow down, but I figured, Who am I to say how

---

Managing Differences in Childrearing Practices

Within yourself . . .

• accept that there are "many right ways" to raise children.

• understand the family's belief systems. Why do parents do what they do? What is their thinking? What are their goals for their child?

• ask for help from parents as you need it. Don't let your frustration build.

• discuss conflicts and alternatives with staff and outside professionals. Get other points of view.

With families . . .

• voice your genuinely held conviction that there are "many right ways" to raise children.

• acknowledge the family's perspective. Understand family circumstances, and share your own.

• help the family to understand your belief system. Why do you do what you do? What are your goals for their child?

• explain that you have to follow practices in group care that you wouldn't necessarily have to follow if you were caring for just one child. Talk about these differences clearly and frequently.

• when you think the parents' way isn't working or they seem to need help, offer it, but don't insist.

• don't make an issue out of every difference. Choose those where you feel negotiation is most vital for the welfare of the child.

• work together to develop respectful consistency for the child. Look for common ground. Find a win-win solution.

With children . . .

• empathize when they have to accommodate many differences.

• make changes in what the child is used to doing gradual.

Many of the language-oriented strategies in the box **Strategies for Bridging Center and Home Cultures** (on page 80) also could be useful.

they should spend their time? Besides, they were performers, and maybe they just had more energy than normal people. They really were fun. We all perked up when they were around, but it seemed like too much for such a small person like Sari. . . .

I finally decided that Sari was going to have to figure out how to cope with them on her own—I couldn't say for certain they were harming her. The best I could do was to offer her a quiet, predictable, "normal" place to rest and to try to see them in a positive light. I think it was the right thing for all of us. Sari's older now, and I know she thrives in all that attention and excitement. Now she joins right in and has a great sense of fun. I guess she had to learn, even as a baby, how to be their child.

This *laissez-faire* approach works when children are not afraid or in any danger. But complicated situations usually require more action on the part of a caregiver. One of the more challenging differences a caregiver faces is parents who encourage her to spank their children. Besides being illegal in many states, spanking brings up a deluge of issues that can send any workshop discussion of childrearing values to

---

Best-Practice Standards and Families' Cultural Expectations

Directors and caregivers may feel torn between the cultural practices and attitudes of the families they serve and best-practice guidelines in the early childhood field (e.g., from NAEYC or Zero to Three). In reality, however, program staff have more decision-making leeway than they often think they do. In specifying and interpreting its accreditation criteria, NAEYC (1998) notes that described practices can be altered or adapted for cultural reasons. For example, accompanying its criterion A-5, which relates to teachers' promotion of children's independence, is the interpretation italicized below:

> A-5. Teachers encourage children's development of independent functioning, as appropriate. Teachers foster the development of age-appropriate self-help skills such as picking up toys, wiping spills, personal grooming (toileting, hand washing), obtaining and caring for materials, and other skills. *(Cultural perspectives of family or community may influence expectations for independence.)* (NAEYC 1998, 68; italics added)

The statement is intended to stress to programs seeking accreditation, as well as to the professionals who make NAEYC's accreditation visits (*validators*), that cultural context should be considered in determining practice. This flexibility is also emphasized in NAEYC's draft updated accreditation criteria now under review (2004).

Not surprisingly, experts differ as to whether such guidelines and standards give sufficient attention to cultural perspectives; some would argue that they do not go far enough in addressing cultural diversity (see, e.g., Hyun 1998; Mallory and New 1994). Moreover, program administrators and staff often do not understand how much room there is for them to adapt child care practices provided they offer a solid rationale for doing so, says Kim Means, NAEYC's senior director for accreditation. When program staff lack this awareness, they feel more constricted than they actually are in the important work of finding solutions to differences in cultural attitudes and preferences.

Relationships, the Heart of Quality Care

run into overtime. One way we have found to help caregivers explore when to cooperate with parental wishes and when to draw the line is to ask themselves these four questions: Is it legal? Does it cause the child pain, humiliation, or harmful restraint? Is this a personal preference, a center policy, a community or cultural norm, or a societal rule? Can I validate either position with sound early care and education research?

Looking at value-based issues from many sides increases empathy and understanding while allowing a response tailored to individual circumstances. Some general strategies for caregivers are outlined in **Managing Differences in Childrearing Practices** (on page 77).

Best practice is culturally sensitive

Many child care centers serve families from cultures that differ from the American mainstream in values, language, and/or childrearing practices. Bicultural and multicultural programs must be sensitive to the expectations and practices of the whole community. A director has to consider how and to what extent to support families' practices if they seem to conflict with best-practice guidelines. How a center approaches child-rearing differences has a big impact on the ability of the adults to form respectful and life-enriching relationships. In a close-knit Hispanic community, the director of a bilingual, bicultural Early Head Start program juggles cultures and expectations. She admits,

> Sometimes I have problems trying to run a culturally sensitive program. . . . If I did everything [the state, accreditation, and other standards] asked me to do, the parents of the children we serve would think we're crazy. For example, the [criteria] encourage children to do things for themselves as early as possible. When they are able to pick up finger food, we're supposed to let them feed themselves. Our families don't expect their children to be independent at an early age. Some parents in my community spoon-feed their children when they are 4 or 5 years old.
>
> I've told my staff to encourage children's independence, but we've had to go at it slowly. I give [the teachers] a lot of leeway because I know they're doing what the parents want them to do. . . . For example, I can't ask my staff to make 2s or 3s clean up after themselves when they spill their milk. If the parents came in and saw the children cleaning tables, they'd say, "What are we paying you for? What's going on in this program!" [In Hispanic culture] cleaning up is a job for adults—not children.

Sometimes, however, the difficulty lies less with the guidelines themselves than in determining when to use the community's approach, when to try new ways, and when to work out cultural "compromises." (NAEYC's accreditation criteria, for example, seek to take cultural differences into account. For more on this, see **Best-Practice Standards and Families' Cultural Expectations.**)

Like others in similar situations, this program's director and caregivers work with standards that sometimes seem removed from the expectations, values, and experiences of the families they serve. And they sometimes choose to follow the families' cultural preferences. When they do implement changes in what children and families are used to, they give themselves plenty of leeway, knowing that staff and families need time to become comfortable doing things differently. When an accreditation observer comes to visit, they explain that they are supporting their families' philosophy and values. It can take courage to present the view that there can be more than one right practice. When program staff show this kind of respect for families, relationships between staff and families become stronger and more authentic.

Strategies for Bridging Center and Home Cultures

Keep families close

• Tape parents' voices to play for a distressed child. Listen together, with the child in your lap.

• Regularly take snapshots of parents and children to share with parents; encourage families to do the same at home. Have a place for children to post their photos in the classroom. Display family pictures, including of caregivers' families. Photographs inspire an exchange of experiences as well as words.

• Encourage families to call the children as often as necessary, especially at first. And allow children to phone their parents as needed for peace of mind.

• Make the classroom a comfortable place and invite families to visit at any time. Ask them to sing songs, tell stories, bring books about their culture to share with the children—and with you.

Make slow, humane transitions

• Encourage families to bring in clothing, food, and personal items for children to hold

and carry, easing the transition between home and child care. Find ways to incorporate the items into center life.

• Watch and mimic the parents' approach to their children.

• Ask parents for ideas that bridge the gap between home and center.

Learn to communicate

• Learn a few words in each child's own language, especially in the first few weeks.

• Listen for the intent of a communication, rather than focusing on halting words of a shy bilingual speaker. Keep in mind that understanding is a work of the heart.

• Make your eyes twinkle with acceptance, allow children and parents time for thinking in two languages, and try to paraphrase without taking over and speaking for the child or parent.

All the general strategies in the previous box **Managing Differences in Childrearing Practices** (on page 77) would apply here too.

For more ideas about collaborating with families in culturally sensitive ways, see **Strategies for Bridging Center and Home Cultures.**

Teachers can be a resource to families

In today's mobile society, with families often living far away from their hometowns, caregivers step into the role that grandparents, aunts, uncles, and neighbors filled in decades past. Their experience makes it easy for many working families to turn to them for wisdom and advice. Most parents care for two or three children, but veteran caregivers with many years on the job may have worked with 50 or more. Experience gives teachers balance, perspective, and common sense when it comes to children's behavior; their assurance and competence puts parents—especially first-timers—at ease. Programs that encourage caregivers to act as resources to families are strengthening strands in the web that joins parents and caregivers in relationship-based care. **How Directors Can Support Caregivers as Resources to Families** (on page 83) offers some places to start.

Help parents transition out of "clock time"

The need for adults to "go to work" does more than physically separate families during certain hours; it sets a pace for their days that is very different from the rhythms of family life. While they are in the workplace, parents are on "clock time"—that is, unless they are ill, they are expected to work quickly and efficiently, to accomplish tasks and meet deadlines in a set time. But the lives of young children have little to do with clock time. Instead, their pace is determined by their developmental stage, abilities, and the ebb and flow of their interest and curiosity. Following a child's lead, it can take more than 30 minutes to walk half a block because the ants patrolling the sidewalk cracks, the pine cone that falls from the tree, and the bees hovering over the grass demand attention.

In high-quality child care, the day's pace is determined by the children, and teachers adjust accordingly. They suspend their adult need for efficiency and instead make sure each child has the time she needs to look through a picture book or make a playdough figure or mail a letter to Mommy. Caregivers learn to pay attention to the small things children notice—the squishiness of the dough, the color of the crayon, the dust floating in a sunbeam. Time isn't measured by the minute and hour hands.

Some parents, at the end of their work days, find it difficult to transition out of clock time. Even when they come home, they don't slow down, just exchange workplace tasks for household chores, and the clock keeps ticking. To parents struggling to keep up with work, home, school, commuting, shopping, and all the rest, it can seem impossible to slow down, much less to go on "toddler time." A caregiver recalls her attitude toward parents picking up their children:

> Before I was a working parent myself, I used to be angry with parents who rushed their children at the end of the day telling them, "Hurry! Put that away! We don't have time for that!" . . . Now I see what work does to a parent.

Another teacher grumbles,

> I always feel badly when parents come to pick up their children and they're in such a rush. It's "Hurry up! We have to get home! Put on your jacket!" . . . I hand them a drawing that the child made that day, and they stuff it into their bag. Because I know how hard the child has worked on that picture, I want to shake the parents and say, "Stop! Pay attention!"

But an experienced teacher can use gentleness and tact to help busy parents reenter their children's world and the slower rhythms of family life. "I remind them of their love for their child and their child's love for them," explains one caregiver. "That calms things down." Another says,

> When parents are in a hurry at pick-up time, they think their children are dawdling, but they aren't—they're just being children. I've talked to hurried parents about making a smoother transition from work to home. I told one parent to visualize her daughter at bedtime with her blanket and her PJs. "Let that picture slow you down." . . . It helped.

When caregivers and parents have caring, trusting relationships, teachers find it easier to feel empathy for harried parents, and parents are open to suggestions without feeling criticized or judged.

Help parents see the big picture

When parents get frustrated or stuck, one of the kindest things a caregiver can do is to act as a sounding board and resource. Veteran caregivers have the long perspective on children's behavior. They know what to do when children spill milk, throw tantrums, bite, or refuse to share. They know which behaviors are worrisome and which are not. Their experience can be a balm to parents who spend a long day at work and come home to behaviors they don't understand or don't know how to cope with. One teacher recalls a baby who cried a lot of the time at the center:

"When parents are in a hurry at pick-up time, they think their children are dawdling, but they aren't— they're just being children."

Relationships, the Heart of Quality Care

How Directors Can Support Caregivers as Resources to Families

With caregivers . . .

• emphasize that their experience with children is a strength.

• encourage their writing notes for families about the day's activities. Parents appreciate ideas on what they can talk about and do with their children at home.

With families . . .

• let them know that caregivers are informed resources, without conveying the impression that they have all the answers or that their way is the *only* way to raise children.

With caregivers and families . . .

• create programs and information-sharing opportunities in which teachers and parents can learn about child development together. This creates a shared vocabulary, common expectations, and a chance to discuss children away from the hurry and scurry of pick-up time.

• provide information on child development as an ongoing educational opportunity for all. Publish a newsletter. Create a family library.

• try an interactive bulletin board with articles, questions that others can respond to, and inspiring quotes for the week. Encourage everyone to participate.

• help everyone draw appropriate distinctions: caregivers are knowledgeable about children in general; parents are the experts on their own children.

> The family was out of sync. When they finished work, they wanted to go home and play with the baby, but the baby wanted to sleep. Then when they were ready for bed, the baby started to cry again. The parents took it hard, because there wasn't much time to be together. . . . I was an extra person to talk to. The parents weren't getting enough sleep, and so we talked about that. I reassured them, "Your child will grow out of this crying: This will pass."

Another caregiver was sitting at a table with a parent one day when two children spilled milk:

> I just told them to clean it up. The parent was more embroiled and upset. For me it was just an ordinary event. . . . I guess I see myself as a buffer. I'm less emotionally involved with the children. I can see the balance. I'm a reality check for parents—a calming or mellowing influence. I comfort parents deliberately and make sure everyone is calm. I let them know it's okay to make mistakes.

Sometimes parents don't realize that their child has entered a new developmental stage until he exhibits unaccustomed behavior, especially if it is troublesome behavior such as tantrums. It can seem that the child has changed overnight. Parents are the experts on their own children, but their experience with the course of development is often limited, especially if they are first-timers. Good caregivers know about the ages and stages of child development and are eager to pass on their knowledge to parents with whom they have a trusting relationship. Here a teacher talks about typical toddler behavior and parental reaction:

> All of a sudden their easygoing child turns stubborn. When a child starts saying no all the time, I tell parents, "That's what 2-year-olds do: They say no!" Parents get it after a while and learn to cope without getting stubborn themselves. . . . I think parents want affirmation from caregivers. They want us to tell them if they're doing something wrong. New parents worry about every detail. I comfort them by telling them they aren't bad people just because they didn't do what the books said. Parents have to learn through trial and error. Children don't come with instructions, and caregivers can help.

◆   ◆   ◆

Follow the lead of your heart

Anyone who has spent time in typical child care centers knows at least one staff member who is that program's heart. Sometimes it is the director, sometimes the cook, sometimes the teacher of the very youngest children. Sometimes it is a determined, friendly, loving parent who leads the center into relationship-based interactions.

A parent we met came to the center to nurse her child several times a day, made easy small talk, took pictures of children and shared them with staff and families, helped caregivers clean up at the end of the day, and organized parent luncheons and weekly pizza parties. It took a while to break through years of formality, but once the ice was broken, warm, responsive adult interactions erupted spontaneously all over the center. Before her child outgrew the center, that mother had attended the wedding of a caregiver, established Friday pizza nights as a regular event, and inspired ongoing staff-parent dialogue. Gifted, loving individuals can make a difference in everyone's life in a child care center, whether the program officially adopts relationship-based care or not. Sometimes one person's influence is so powerful that the climate changes and relationship-based care becomes the norm organically, rather than by policy.

Still, we can do more. System-wide organizational changes can ensure that everyone enjoys the benefits of relationship-based care. Centers around the country are introducing policies that support and protect relationships and give them room to take root and flourish. **Chapters 4 and 5** look at such practices.

4

Setting Policies to Meet Children's Needs

Relationship-based care is the best way to meet the needs of young children, wherever they spend their days. So the challenge for child care centers is not whether relationship-based care should be a priority but how to make it so. But what can a program do when the needs of children seem in direct conflict with fiscal constraints? Best practice is good for children, but it can be expensive. Are there policy changes that can be implemented at little cost? What about workplace norms that seem to meet the needs of parents, caregivers, and directors but are detrimental to young children? How do we bring about shifts in practice to meet children's developmental needs when decision makers see other priorities as more pressing?

Sometimes the gap between the ideal and what is feasible looks too great; a more limited approach seems to be the only solution. But as early care and education researcher Ellen Galinsky frequently reminded the field at conferences and meetings we attended in the 1990s, "You pay now or you pay later." If the early care and education profession doesn't make the needs of children a high priority, we all will suffer the consequences down the road.

Fortunately, plenty of leaders are already blazing the trail. A surprising number of innovative centers have assessed the situation, weighed the possibilities, and made relationship-based care their goal. Their commitment and enthusiasm inspired us to look more deeply at the steps they have taken along the way. What changes in policies and practices did they make? What's now in place? Are there any drawbacks? Are caregiver-child-parent connections actually stronger? How do the programs cover any added cost? What obstacles to implementation did they encounter, and how did they overcome them? What can their experiences teach us?

The list of five strategies in this chapter grew out of our observations and conversations with staff and families at innovative centers. Their stories led us to conclude that implementing a program of relationship-based care depends less on money than on vision, planning, and patient teamwork. More often than not, it is a persistent determination to put children's needs first that makes the difference. In most of the programs, change began with a few people who were as dedicated to their caring relationships with one another as they were determined to meet the children's needs. Individual attitudes and belief in the importance of relationships, as described in **Chapter 3,** lay the groundwork. Acting on that belief to shape policy and practice makes relationship-based care a reality.

Strategy #1: Low ratios and small group sizes

Ratio, the number of caregivers to children, and *group size,* the total number of children in a room—along with caregiver experience and training—have been used for decades by the early care and education profession as indicators of quality of care. These numbers help predict the amount of warm, responsive attention that each child is likely to receive from caregivers in a given setting. The younger or more dependent the children, the more important low ratios, small group sizes, and caregiver expertise become.

State licensing laws regulate the maximum numbers allowed for safety; professional standards address the numbers recommended for quality. Nature's laws set a benchmark. A human mother usually gives birth to one, maybe two, babies at a time, at least a year apart. Although we all know parents and caregivers who nurture a number of children at once, and do it well, we also know that the very best we can do for the youngest child is still one-to-one. As children grow more verbal and independent and their needs become more predictable and easier to manage, somewhat higher ratios and larger group sizes are more realistic. However, bigger is not better at any age when it comes to nurturing human beings. Lower numbers are a good place to start when child-centered, relationship-based care is the goal. (See **About Ratios and Group Sizes.**)

Benefits of low ratios and small group sizes

For children. Children of all ages benefit from low staff-child ratios and small group sizes; small numbers are critical for children under 3 and those with special needs. Numbers affect the caregivers' ability to balance individualized time and attention with the realities of group care. Children in programs with low ratios and small groups can get their physical and emotional needs met without having to compete or wait for too many others to have their turn. They are more likely to experience warm, responsive adult relationships because the caregivers aren't spread so thin that they lose sight of individual children and see only a herd in need of control.

When each caregiver has responsibility for a smaller number of children, routines can be adjusted to individual rhythms, rather than regulated by the clock. Caregivers are tuned in. They don't have to refer to a schedule to know when it's time for diaper changes. They

---

About Ratios and Group Sizes

What the experts recommend:

• [AAP, APHA, NRCHSCC] The recommended staff-child ratio for children birth to 12 months is 1:3 with a maximum group size of six. For children 13–30 months, the recommendation is 1:4 with a group size of eight. For 31–35 months, it is 1:5 with a group size of 10. (American Academy of Pediatrics, American Public Health Association, & National Resource Center for Health and Safety in Child Care 2002, 4)

• [Zero to Three] "Empirical research and the wisdom of early care specialists have consistently identified these two indicators as critical to quality child care. No more than six children who are not yet mobile should be in a group: a caregiver should be responsible for no more than three young infants. . . . For children 18 months to 3 years, group size should be no more than 12, staff-to-child ratios, 1:4." (Lally et al. 1995, 32)

• [NAEYC] "Smaller group sizes and larger numbers of staff to children are related to positive outcomes for children. . . . Multiage grouping is both permissible and desirable. When no infants are included, the staff-child ratio and group size requirements shall be based on the age of the majority of the children in the group. When infants are included, ratios and group size for infants must be maintained. . . . Maximum group size is determined by the distribution of ages in the group. Group size limitations will vary depending on the type of activity, whether it is indoors or outdoors; the inclusion of children with special needs; and other factors." (NAEYC 1998b, 45–48)

Recognizing the complexity of accounting for all these factors, NAEYC offers its guidance in the form of a table, "Recommended Staff-Child Ratios within Group Size" (1998b, 47). For the youngest children, NAEYC's recommendations more or less parallel those of Zero to Three.

The current status in the states:

• Only four states—Hawaii, Kansas, Massachusetts, Maryland—have a 1:3 staff-infant ratio. Thirty-three states have a 1:4 ratio. (Children's Foundation 2003)

---

have time to read a story or rock a fussy baby to sleep. It's easier to let a toddler dawdle on the potty or coax a shy child to join small-group play. With only four toddlers to care for, a caregiver can laugh at silly bread and bean play at lunch; he can let the children's individual paces guide the flow into naptime. Each child is recognized and valued as part of "the family," rather than shuffled like an object in an anonymous crowd.

Lower ratios and smaller group sizes decrease the noise level, reduce confusion, and enhance group dynamics in a classroom. The flow of activity is quieter and more orderly, especially at transition times. For example, in one Georgia center we observed, the teachers divided a classroom of 20 young 3-year-olds into two groups of 10 each. Each group spent the whole day with one of the classroom's two caregivers, except during free time, when all 20 used the entire room to play. This classroom functioned more smoothly than others we observed with two caregivers and the same number of children in one large group. In the divided groups, evidence of bonding was plentiful between children and their special adults.

However, the benefits of splitting one large group into two smaller ones were not apparent to the staff at that center. It was difficult to convince anyone there that the children were actually better off in the arrangement. When the caregivers were complimented, they were surprised. They had divided up the classroom space and the larger group simply because they disliked each other and found it hard to work together. These teachers were considered "poor at teamwork" by their director, and everyone looked at the situation through that filter.

With such a narrow focus, this center missed the fact that small numbers keep life relaxed; the need for management and coordination is less, even between teammates. When children are kept in small groups with low ratios, behavior challenges are less frequent, less intense, and easier to handle. Each child comes to believe "I count!" Because they get individualized attention, the children see themselves as lovable and worthy of that attention; their experiences tell them that life is full of thoughtful adults who will meet their needs and keep them safe. No one *prefers* to be herded. Whether you are 6 months old or 60 years old, it is important to be individually known—and loved.

For families. When classroom numbers are low, drop-off and pick-up times are smoother and less hurried. The room feels like a home instead of a busy train station. Relationships with caregivers can develop more easily and naturally. Family members and caregivers are likely to start real conversations and come to know each other as

> No one *prefers* to be herded. Whether you are 6 months old or 60 years old, it is important to be individually known—and loved.

individuals. Parents also get to know one another and begin to recognize that they are part of a small community that cares.

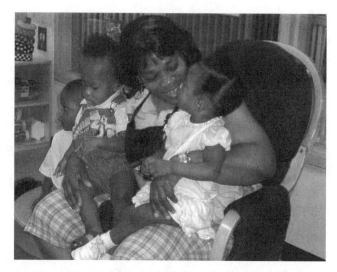

For caregivers. Caregivers thrive when numbers are low because smaller groups of children are more manageable—it is that simple. With fewer children it is easier to get to know and be responsive to each child. There is less of a need for assembly-line care, less of a temptation to put children off, less necessity to juggle one child's need against another's. As in a small family or a family child care home, routines evolve naturally and are flexible. There are fewer mouths to feed, fewer diapers to change, fewer backs to rub at naptime. Rainy days when children can't go out to play or days spent with substitutes don't feel like nightmares. Caregivers have more time to see children and parents as individuals who are worth getting to know, and that makes the job more enjoyable and satisfying. There is less burnout, less chaos, less stress. Given the choice, who would insist on caring for *more* children rather than fewer?

For directors and centers. Many directors run from trying to balance the benefit of low numbers and their center's fiscal needs. But we believe that those who find ways to decrease ratios and group sizes within a workable budget will never regret the effort. Low numbers make it easier for a program to become accredited and to maintain high standards of warm, responsive care. Centers feel homier and make a good impression on families. Even in large centers, when each classroom is a small oasis of ongoing, satisfying relationships a sense of quality pervades the whole.

Low numbers allow even new caregivers to manage children's needs with minimal stress, and that means fewer children (and caregivers) out of control. Workplace conditions are reasonable, so directors worry less about burnout, turnover, and training staff to survive.

Moving toward low ratios and small group sizes

One veteran director made numbers her first priority when she took a new job five years ago:

We were able to afford it, so when I became the director, I reduced our enrollment from 120 to 70. We have five classes and seven teachers. It really makes a difference! I know every single child. I don't think the parents appreciate or even understand what we've done—until they move to another [larger] center. We just did it because it was the right thing to do.

Lowering its overall size made this center feel more human and rich in relationships. Understanding the importance of relationships between teachers and directors and each family and child is critical. Unless relationships are given first priority, change is nearly impossible. Opposition to lowering the numbers can be fierce, because financial considerations are real. When relationships come first, such change is possible.

A long-time Georgia early childhood advocate agrees that the conversation must move beyond *whether* to lower numbers to *how* to reduce them. As her story below indicates, sometimes the starting point is removing the option of large numbers altogether.

> In 1974 the Georgia legislature was ignorantly voting in favor of high ratios and large group sizes because they felt it would be "less of a shock" when young children entered elementary school—can you imagine? The legal infant ratio was 1:7 and the group size allowed was 14. In a lot of centers the babies stayed in their cribs most of every day, except when harried caregivers let a few at a time down on the floor to practice crawling or walking. Toddler ratios allowed 1:9; the 2-year-old ratios were 1:12. As many as three toddler groups per room were permitted, depending on space. The rooms were unbelievably loud and full of fussiness. Children were obviously getting poor-quality care, but the private, for-profit [child care] lobby was focused on survival. They helped maintain high ratios and large groups for several more years, claiming that lower numbers would "put everyone out of business."
>
> Finally we were able to use NAEYC's standards to educate our legislature, and we pressured them into dropping the numbers. Our slogan was, "Two arms can't hold seven babies." We only got it down to one less child for each age group, with smaller group sizes all around; but we felt like that was a big victory at the time. You cannot imagine the hoopla over that small change. But because they had no choice, most centers found ways to meet these lower ratios and group sizes. Thanks to NAEYC accreditation and Early Head Start, there are now some [centers] that have voluntarily moved to much better ratios and group sizes. The difference [in those classrooms] is amazing!

Think how, not whether. Few adults *prefer* to manage very young children in very large groups. Resistance to small numbers largely stems from concern for center finances. But there are various strategies for addressing those issues. Some centers begin charging more for infant and toddler care. Others charge a flat rate for all ages, so the less-expensive preschool classrooms can carry the more-expensive baby rooms. Whatever strategy they choose, center administrators and governing boards must make a firm decision and be willing to risk losing some parents (and therefore income), at least at first. High ratios and large groups might seem like good business, but packing early childhood classrooms to capacity and hiring fewer caregivers is short-sighted policy that puts young children at risk. A clear, persistent message is necessary for change. Administrators have to be convinced that low numbers and relationship-based care are what's best in the long run for everyone—and for the viability of the center.

This change in perspective can take time. In one well-respected center that was eager to improve quality, the administrators were surprised when they were asked by their consultant to look at their infant and toddler rooms through the lens of relationships. Until then they had naively assumed that big groups were more "fun" for children and "safer." They took a chance and reduced group sizes, so that their classrooms never had more than eight children under age 3. They saw an immediate and obvious reward of increased quality and deeper relationships.

Many centers have found creative, reasonable approaches to lowering ratios and group sizes. One Georgia program used doors with clear plastic panels and half-walls to divide a large room in two. Each side had a class of 10 toddlers and two caregivers. These groups were further divided into two sets of five children and one teacher each, a ratio of 1:5. To maintain staff relationships and to make break-coverage work, teachers slid the doors open at naptime and during free-play times. This center's successful results inspired several others to do the same. When the program took on an Early Head Start contract and a commitment to a ratio of 1:4, it was an easy solution to reduce the numbers once more, to the required maximum of eight children and two adults.

Use volunteers and interns for extra arms and laps and to improve ratios. In parent cooperatives and some center classrooms, family volunteering is required as a way of reducing staff ratios and adding fresh perspectives. As a side benefit, parents get to know the other children and parents—offering still more connections for everyone, especially when the relationships grow to extend beyond the classroom. Some centers also welcome interns or foster grandparents. For example, with support from a local senior citizens project, The Sheltering Arms, Inc., child care system in Atlanta invites community

The role of
the *abuelas*
("grandmothers")
depends on the
personality of
the volunteer
and the needs of
the classroom.

grandparents to commit to regular hours, making it possible for many classrooms to have at least one helper on a predictable schedule. Their relationships with children and staff are consistent; if they are around at drop-off or pick-up time, they also get to know parents.

The foster grandparents work with the caregivers as effective supports, not just as additional warm bodies. Some prefer to do chores and free up the teachers to be with their groups; others are companions to the children in the book area, at the puzzle tables, or wherever else they are needed. Children get to know them one-on-one. When a child feels sleepy or out of sorts, he seeks out a nurturing grandparent's lap. We were particularly impressed with a 70-something woman, whom the children called Grand-Betty. She brought her favorite upbeat CDs and danced with the children every morning while the caregivers of these older 2-year-olds gathered materials for small-group time. Together, she and the teachers created an effective, enthusiastic team.

At bilingual, bicultural Ibero Early Childhood Services, in Rochester, New York, Spanish-speaking seniors can sign up for a morning or an afternoon shift with infants, toddlers, or preschoolers. As in the Sheltering Arms program, the role of the *abuelas* ("grandmothers") depends on the personality of the volunteer and the needs of the classroom. Some like to mop and clean up after snacks; some like to run errands, going to the kitchen or the office as needed. Some like to sit with the preschool children when they're doing table projects to offer help, praise, or simple companionship. Now and then they take a distressed child out for a walk around the center, to see what the other children and adults are doing.

The center doesn't recruit the *abuelas* for the purpose of improving staff-child ratios, but that is an obvious benefit. Instead, they free the regular caregivers to have more one-on-one time with the children. The *abuelas* represent the extended family tradition that is so important in the upbringing of Latino children in that community. The staff members welcome the help; parents like the idea that elders from the neighborhood are there to look after their children; and the children enjoy the extra love and ready smiles and hugs.

Hire support staff for flexible assignment. Some centers reduce ratios by hiring staff part-time and as floaters to rotate among several classrooms and cover during breaks and absences. In small centers the director or cook may play this floater role as needed or on a regular basis. As children get to know these helpers, especially if they come at predictable times each day, the children have less adjustment when their regular caregivers are out.

Strategy #2: Primary caregiving

Primary caregiving means that the infant or toddler and his family have someone special with whom to build an intimate relationship (Lally et al. 1995). From the time a child enters the program, the parent knows who is principally responsible for that child's care. In the last 10 years primary caregiving has been widely promoted for children birth to age 3 by Early Head Start, WestEd, and Zero to Three.

A primary caregiver is responsible for a particular, small group of children within the classroom. She doesn't have the full complement of decision-making rights that parents do, and she cannot completely ignore the needs of children in other groups in the room. But inside those limits, a primary caregiver attends completely to the needs of the children in her group. She changes their diapers, helps them with the potty and hand washing, offers comforting words, feeds them bottles, and sits with them at the table for meals. She sets up predict-able expectations for interactions between herself and the children in her group; she determines which skills and manners seem appropriate for their ages and cultural backgrounds. She plans their learning activities, does regular observations, documents progress, and shares anecdotes on their development with their families. **It's Primary Caregiving If…** (on page 94) lists some ways to determine what is happening in a classroom.

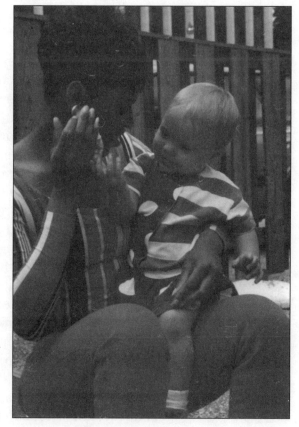

Because the primary caregiver is focused on a certain group of children, she is more likely to bond with them, and her bond tends to be deeper than if she shared equal responsibility with coworkers for the group as a whole. She is more likely to learn how to interpret each child's cues and respond to each child's particular needs in sensitive, developmentally appropriate ways. She knows that Patty hates to be hurried and that Simon usually fusses when he wakes up from his nap. She remembers that Elizabeth hates peas and that Mohid's family doesn't eat pork. Her care is warm, responsive, and individual. For their part, the children in her group are more likely to bond with her, and their bonds tend to be deeper as well.

It's Primary Caregiving If . . .

Individual children . . .

• notice what their caregiver is doing through the day; notice and react to her arrivals and departures from the room.

• often prefer to be with their caregiver when given a choice.

• know their caregiver's name.

Caregivers . . .

• provide for daily nurturing routines for the children in their own small groups—meals and snacks, diaper changes or toilet routines, naptime settling, small-group activity times.

• have special one-on-one times with each child in their group each day—lap reading, making eye contact, smiling, calling child's name now and then, sharing nuzzles, hugging, snuggling, holding, talking and singing at child's eye level, and sharing

interactive, learning experiences with individual children.

Families . . .

• know that the same caregiver keeps track of their child and what the child does each day.

• know that the same caregiver plans for their child's learning activities, observes the child in the small group, keeps anecdotal records on their child's developmental progress, and both formally and informally shares her observations of their child.

• see a list of names of each small group posted prominently for them.

• see pictures of each small group displayed prominently for children, families, and staff.

• are referred pleasantly to the same caregiver, whenever they ask staff at the center about their child.

Because primary caregiving is a matter of internal organization rather than increasing staff, it pays huge dividends for little or no additional expense and is easy for a center to implement. Some caregiver teams simply divide their class into smaller groups and each adult assumes the primary responsibility for a few of the children. In some programs the director assigns the adults to certain children in the room; in still others, a child informally chooses the person she feels closest to, creating primary caregiving based on the child's own preferences.

Even though a classroom is divided into smaller, primary caregiving groups, a lead caregiver can still be responsible for overall organization and planning. Teachers are expected to work together as a team and help all the children. But there is an obvious, observable, *special* relationship between each small group of children and their special adult. The children know their primary caregiver's name; the parents seek her out. Children in a class may gather a few times a day for appropriate large-group activities, but *more* of their time is spent in their small nesting group with their same regular caregiver, especially for nurturing routines.

The model for primary caregiving relationships is home or family child care, not school. Here's how one center describes it:

One way to look at primary caregiving is that caregivers are like sisters who share a house. Each [sister] has [her own] small family of children; the other [children in the house] are her nieces and nephews—her sisters' children. Everyone works together to make the home work; but when a child needs "Mommy," everyone—especially the child—knows who that special adult is, and they all help the child find her. Relationships are valued in primary caregiving; the daily game of "musical adults" is minimal.

Benefits of these small "families" are great, no matter how long they remain together over time.

Benefits of primary caregiving

For children. The deep attachment that children form with their primary caregiver gives them the security and emotional support they need for healthy development. Children's eyes light up when their caregiver walks into the room—just as they do when the children's parent comes in—and the children notice when their caregiver leaves. She is the one these children turn to if they are out of sorts or need a hug. They hide behind her and peek around her legs when strangers enter the room. If they are hurt or tired or scared or need a diaper change, she is the one they look for first. The children know their special caregiver the way children know their parents. They know when she is in a playful mood and when she is feeling stressed. They know how she reacts to spilt milk or tantrums and what she expects from them when they make a mistake. This intimate understanding of her as a person allows the children to get beyond survival and focus on loving and learning.

Having a primary caregiver makes a child's world feel predictable and inspires confidence. Primary caregiving ensures that every child in the program has an advocate—a special person who knows a lot about that child's personality, development, and family members. This primary caregiving assignment gives each child a chance to form an intimate and secure bond, a secure base from which he can explore the world (Lally 1995).

The benefits of a relationship with a primary caregiver are similar to the benefits of a relationship with a loving and responsive parent. Children are less likely to feel overwhelmed and frustrated, are quicker to settle down, and are more patient when they have to wait for help. As one astute caregiver explains,

> It's easy to think of babies as people without any personality, but that isn't true. They're all different. Some like to be held lying down and some like to be up against your chest. Some fuss to feed themselves and some

"One way to look at primary caregiving is that caregivers are like sisters who share a house."

are happy being fed. If you respond to children as individuals they come to trust you. They are slower to cry and throw tantrums, because they know someone—you—will listen and respond to their need.

Everyday interactions between very young children and a caregiver attuned to their unique cues help children develop a positive sense of self. A consistent, caring adult who has had time and opportunity to understand a child will know whether he is mellow or intense. She knows his current interests—the mirror, his toes, the climbing cushions, the ball with the bells inside. She can read the child's emotions and knows whether he can wait or is about to collapse in despair. That she is so attuned teaches the child that he is safe, listened to, and understood. Her responses teach him that what he does is important; he has an impact on the people around him. The child learns that the world can be trusted and that if he needs help or comfort, someone special will be there to take care of him.

A primary caregiver also is more likely to know about each child's life at home. The primary caregiving bond makes the important adults in the child's life more inclined to share information, develop a relationship with each other, and work together to meet the child's needs. This helps a primary caregiver be aware of circumstances that affect a child's behavior. When the child is cranky, his primary caregiver is more likely to know that it is because the family had weekend company or that he may have caught his sister's cold.

For families. Because the primary caregiver knows each child in her group so well, she can share each child's discoveries, interests, and frustrations with that family. With only a limited number of families to focus on, a primary caregiver is more likely to form connections with each family naturally and authentically. When a specific adult is clearly identified for the job of caring for their child, parents may find it easier to open themselves to partnership. As in family child care homes, where providers work with the same families over time, adults in primary caregiving programs are more motivated to develop and sustain relationships with each other.

Further, when classrooms are organized into primary caregiving groups, families know which caregiver to turn to when they have a concern or question. Close parent-caregiver relationships lessen the predictable anxiety parents have about leaving their children in the hands of strangers. Primary caregiving arrangements help parents lower their defenses, as they begin to trust that there is one special caregiver in the classroom who has the best interests of their specific child at heart.

Caregivers who have worked in settings with and without primary caregiving attest to its benefits.

For caregivers. Like low ratios and small group sizes, primary caregiving arrangements make children's behavior easier to predict and manage, which means that caregivers are more likely to look forward to seeing those children day after day. Primary care assignments allow caregivers to get to know the children's families in genuine ways. Relationships tend to be mutually supportive and long lasting; they become a perk and an incentive to stay on the job. Primary caregiving also reduces the potential for conflict with coworkers. Because it is clear who is primarily responsible for which child, tensions are reduced between coworkers over such issues as whose turn it is to cope with difficult children.

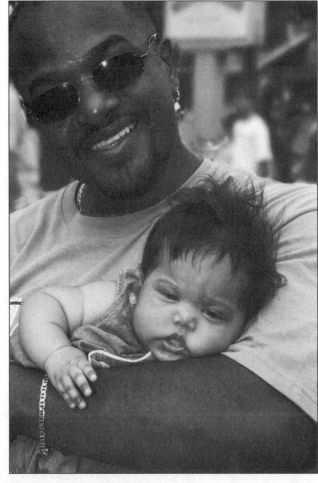

Caregivers who have worked in settings with and without primary caregiving attest to its benefits. Early in her career, one of us (Lynn) took a job as primary caregiver for 15 preschoolers. She shared a large room with two other primary caregivers and their groups of 4-year-olds. Each group had a special space in the larger room that was their niche for most of the day. This is where the group ate family-style, napped together, and enjoyed their small-group learning activities. Two or three times a day the whole room was opened to all 45 children for free play or for short community-building activities such as sing-a-longs, introduction of concepts, or movies. The primary caregiving groups were large by some standards, but each caregiver felt a genuine sense of family with her children. Lynn stayed three and a half years—and even moved up with one group. Decades later she can still name many of her children. She remains in touch with a few families and is greeted joyously by others when she sees them now and then around town.

In contrast, she later worked in a more typical setting of three caregivers, 45 preschoolers, and no primary caregiving assignments. The program was respected nationally, but the care felt impersonal to her, more institutional than family-like. The 4-year-olds were taught, fed, moved, and napped in one large group or broken up arbitrarily by adult whim into smaller ones. The lead caregiver did most of the "teaching," while Lynn and a second assistant did more of the chores. At mealtime, children had to wait, their hands in their laps, until all 45 were served. The center's director handled relationships with families, and caregivers were asked to limit their interactions with parents to brief hellos and good-byes. Lynn lasted six months and cannot remember one child or even the names of her team members.

For directors and centers. When primary caregiving is in place, a center feels calm and settled. Relationships are stronger, and predictable expectations reduce confusion, tantrums, and tears. It is clear who is responsible for which children. It is also safer, because bonded caregivers are more likely to pay attention to their children and anticipate their behavior. With primary caregiving, teachers must meet the needs of one specific group of children instead of exhausting themselves trying to cover everyone's needs, everywhere, all day long. As with low numbers, primary caregiving improves workplace conditions for caregivers; burnout is less common and directors are more likely to retain staff.

Moving toward primary caregiving

Remember from **Chapter 2** the chaotic classroom of 1- and 2-year-olds being yelled at to "Use your spoon!" Here is what happened when primary caregiving is introduced:

At their director's request, Miss Mathews, Mrs. Lee, and Miss Threadgood agree to be mentored for six months as primary caregivers, with the shared goals of reducing lunchtime chaos and raising the overall quality of care in their room. The teachers get together and decide which children and caregivers are most comfortable together, and create new groups of four toddlers each. Changes come slowly. When time or patience gets away from them, they revert back to their old ways, with each of them focusing on all 12 children, assembly-line routines, and the lead teacher barking orders at everyone. It takes at least three weeks for them to learn to concentrate on their own group exclusively. It takes several more weeks for them to feel comfortable spending most of their time in small groups.

Group management and behavior problems begin dropping away. The children still share the entire room during choice time, play outside as a whole class, and sing in a large group circle each day. But each child's daily story circles and nurturing routines occur with the primary caregiver and the same group of three classmates. The small groups eat together, listen to stories together, and nap near one another in their "nest" area. Miss Mathews admires Mai Le when she twirls in her new dress, instead of hurrying her onto the potty. David's puzzle skills strike Mrs. Lee as brilliant, instead of an irritation that delays lunch. The room feels more like a home. The teachers start having real conversations with the children in their group; they notice small, quiet, individual needs—a drippy nose, untied shoes, a requested CD.

Evidence of bonding appears. Children brighten up when their special teacher arrives. They seek her out when they have a boo-boo or need a diaper change. The teachers still look out for the other children, but they know the children in their own group best. Each child has a special adult to turn to when comfort is needed.

Imagine the difference at lunchtime! The children have to learn only one adult's routine. The "spoon-sensitive" Mrs. Lee finally reaps success, because the bonds she has developed with her children make them more interested in meeting her particular expectations. At the chatty Miss Mathews's table, her children learn to use their spoons by watching her, safe from sudden chastisement. The table-hopping Miss Threadgood struggles the longest, but once she is sitting still long enough to notice her children's individual personalities and needs, their food-smearing antics disappear.

By the end of the six months all three teachers are hooked on primary caregiving. "I can't imagine why we were working so hard!" one says. Parents love the change too. They know which teacher to talk to, and can develop a meaningful relationship with her, knowing she is the caregiver who spends the most time with their child.

> "[With primary caregiving in place,] group management and behavior problems begin dropping away."

As beneficial as primary caregiving is for children, teachers, and families, transitioning to it surfaces predictable obstacles.

"What if I'm stuck with the caregiver from hell?" Every director knows a child or parent who is troublesome or a caregiver who rubs some people the wrong way. People don't always get along, and sometimes it is no one's fault. Problems may be the result of insufficient bonding or a sense among the adults that the relationship is not worth the effort to fix. Policies that address caregiver-child and parent-caregiver mismatches are a must. When primary caregiving is the way and the match is right, adults are helped to connect in respectful ways, and everyone works to develop problem-solving skills. Rather than cause problems, primary caregiving helps adults create good matches and adjust to poor ones.

Allowing parents, children, and caregivers to help select one another is a good match-making strategy. So too is deciding in advance how to cope with the inevitable conflicts. It makes sense to have a process for reporting grievances that outlines steps for working things out. When adults know they will get the time and guidance it takes to work through interpersonal issues, they generally will work harder and more constructively. One teacher admits,

> I am actually closest to the children and families I have had to struggle with to make things work. It's like a marriage or a family. If you give up, things never get resolved, and you usually end up in the same place with the next one.

"What if the children become *too* attached?" Mention primary caregiving in some centers and you'll hear this kind of resistance from parents as well as staff. What if children become so attached to the primary caregiver that they are distraught or difficult to manage when he goes on vacation or leaves the room? Parents also worry that their child will love the caregiver more than them, will want to see the caregiver at night and on the weekends, and won't want to leave child care at the end of the day. Strong attachments in child care can make parents feel jealous and guilty ("If I had stayed home with Becca, *I* would be the one getting all those hugs and kisses"). Children *do* become attached to the adults who care for them—that's one of the goals of primary caregiving. We wouldn't want children *not* to care when their parents leave; a certain amount of separation anxiety is healthy—a sign of attachment. The same is true of a bonded relationship between a child and a primary caregiver.

Caregiving teams who make children's attachment needs a priority learn to manage the separations. One caregiver explains,

> It's *true* we form close attachments to children—that's part of our job. But we also have to teach children to say good-bye. People leave children's lives all the time. Mothers go to the store, mothers go to work. Caregivers go to the bathroom, caregivers go on vacation. We teach children that it can be hard to say good-bye to people you love, but it's natural and something you have to learn to do.

According to such caregivers, attachment makes life easier instead of more difficult. At one center a teacher recalls,

> I was worried that the children would become too attached to my coworkers or me if we switched to primary caregiving. I didn't want children crying every time my coworker walked out of the room. Primary caregiving *did* make the children more attached, but it was a lot easier to deal with than before. I could say, "I know you miss Eileen, but she'll be back in a few minutes." Or I could say, "I know you love Eileen, and she loves you."
>
> Before, we talked about children's attachments, but we didn't take them seriously and we didn't talk about them with the children. When we became primary caregivers, it was as though we gave children permission to attach. We recognized that those bonds were important and it was okay for us to talk about them.

"When we became primary caregivers, it was as though we gave children permission to attach."

In the following teacher's experience, once children connect to one primary caregiver, they become more attached to *all* the adults in the room:

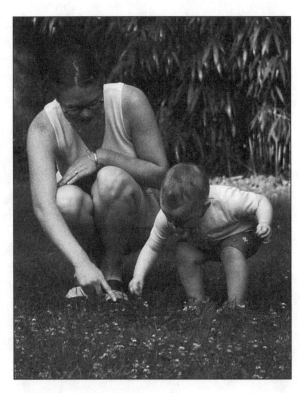

> We expected the children would be more attached when we became primary caregivers, but our fears were exaggerated. Miss Francine's children *were* closer to her than to me, but I was closer to her children than I'd been before, too. . . . They knew they weren't abandoned when Francine left, because I called to them, distracted them. They felt sad, but they knew I understood their feelings, and I was still there.
>
> I think relationships with primary caregivers are a lot like relationships in a family at home. Children have favorites at home too. Most young children prefer their mothers, and they feel sad when their mothers go away. But if their dads or their grandmas are there, they will go to them for comfort and feel safe in their arms. The child's relationships with his mother and father and grandma are all different, but other people can substitute for the mother and it's all right.

Caregivers in the San Diego area told us that the positives of primary caregiving outweigh the negatives, no matter how distressing the separations are. Here's what two of them said:

> Separations are hard. My coworker went on vacation, and some of the children missed her quite a bit. We spent a lot of time talking about where she went and when she was coming back. We made a strip calendar and cut off the days so they could tell how much time was left until she'd be here again. We got through it.

> There is a special, intimate feeling in our classroom. We get to know each child and each family personally in a way we couldn't before when we were responsible for everyone in the room. It's so much more satisfying. I'd never go back to the old way, no matter how much one of the children missed Mary when she left the room.

Most of the parents we talked to agree. Here's a typical story:

> I used family child care before I came here; I didn't trust centers. Most of them are too impersonal. But here, it's different. Maria is Paulo's caregiver; she really knows my child and she knows me too. She is the one who sees what he did during the day and she can tell me if I ask. I have friends who pick their children up at centers, and the only thing they hear about is the number of diaper changes and what their children had for lunch. They

don't know what their children played with or who their friends are. Maria can tell me anything I want to know. The other day she told me he was watching himself in the mirror. She notices things like that. Sure, my son will miss Maria when she goes on vacation—he misses her on the weekend! But that's good news to me. I want him to love his caregiver. We can put up with vacations.

Primary caregiving makes all the difference to the comfort level of anxious parents.

Strategy #3: Continuity of care

The practice of *continuity of care* means keeping a group of children and their caregiver together until preschool—or beyond. The children in the group can be all the same age or mixed, but planning and managing this strategy is easier for the center when ages are mixed. In contrast, traditional centers group infants and toddlers narrowly by age in classrooms staffed and equipped for their developmental stage. As they grow, the children must change caregivers and rooms, "moving up" from the Young Infant Room to the Mobile Infant Room to the Toddler Room and so on, as often as every six to eight months, depending on enrollment and other circumstances. These changes force children, caregivers, and families to rebuild trust and confidence again and again, as the child goes through the program.

The difference is dramatic between classrooms where relationships are routinely broken and rooms where they are kept intact. At one center during the moving-up cycle we noticed two classrooms that seemed settled and calm compared with the chaos and confusion around them. Why no fuss? The caregivers, with a mixture of relief and satisfaction, explained that they were remaining with their children for the coming year. In their classrooms, instead of triggering an avalanche of change, life and learning were permitted to continue without disruption.

At that center, chance programming gave stability to those lucky few. Centers that offer continuity of care keep children with one or more of the same caregivers as a matter of policy. Some centers group children broadly by age, caring for children birth–18 months or older in the same classroom and moving them and their caregiving team to a new room at the end of the year. Others group children more narrowly by age. Either way, the caregivers and the children remain together when the group moves up. The goal of a continuity policy is to permit deep and secure attachments to develop between children and their

> "We get to know each child and each family personally in a way we couldn't before when we were responsible for everyone in the room."

caregivers and to encourage warm relationships between the children's significant adults. It is particularly important for infants and toddlers, who at that age are developing an identity and need strong attachments for healthy brain development.

> Losing [a beloved caregiver] . . . at the end of the first year because . . . a baby must graduate from the baby room into the toddler room is not what any of us would prescribe for a baby trying to grow emotionally in a healthy way. Would we deliberately recommend changing mothers every year? (Greenspan 2001, 220)

According to leaders in the field of infant/toddler care such as Zero to Three and WestEd, young children should stay with the same caregiver for their first three years of life (Lally et al. 1995; PITC 1997). In this ideal, a bonded group of children and their caregiving team move together when they change rooms, or they spend all three years in the same room if the space is large enough and meets other state requirements. After they have turned 3, the children move up together to preschool, and the caregiving team "loops back" for another "rotation" with a new group of children.

Another way of providing continuity is to move one of the familiar caregivers from a team with the children when they change rooms. This strategy doesn't permit children to have a continuous relationship with the entire caregiving team, but they do remain with at least one trusted and familiar adult. This approach is sometimes regarded as a first step for centers that are moving toward full continuity of care.

Benefits of continuity of care

For children. In many ways, the relationships in programs that offer continuity of care resemble those of high-quality family child care or nanny care. Because the children and caregivers stay together so long, they become deeply attached to each other. The caregivers see and respond to their children as individuals. Caregivers have time to bond with parents too, so they are familiar with each family's childrearing style. They know what's happening day to day in the child's life outside the center and are aware of important events that affect the child and the family.

Caregivers we spoke to from the University of New Mexico Children's Campus for Early Care and Education and from Grossmont College Child Care, where continuity of care is an established part of both programs, are enthusiastic about the benefits to children. Says one,

"Would we deliberately recommend changing mothers every year?"

Continuity of care frees children from stresses that prevent them from learning. Children who have to cope with numerous transitions to new rooms, new caregivers, new room arrangements, and new styles of interacting have to spend energy figuring out the rules and expectations of the new setting. It's stressful and energy consuming. Children who have continuity of care aren't as caught up in the logistics or mechanics of change. They're free to do the things that are natural to their age—walking, climbing, standing, and communicating.

A veteran caregiver believes that children who stay with the same caregivers from infancy are less aggressive and easier to manage when they turn 2 years old (children enter her classroom at 24–34 months).

> I've come to think that the toddler year is easier on the children and the caregivers when there is continuity of care. The caregivers have been with a child for a year and already know how to read her cues. They don't provoke problems or balkiness through their own fumbling. . . . I don't have evidence to document this, but I think there is less toilet regression, biting, and aggression when children stay with the same caregivers. When children have to make many changes, they are more concerned with trust and relationships because [those things] aren't a given. Aggressive behavior is more pronounced.

"Consistency of care has reduced [my son's] stress level and made him easier to care for."

A caregiver who works with children with disabilities is convinced that continuity enables her to provide better care. She says,

> It's always hard to raise the subject of developmental delays with parents. They're afraid for their children and themselves when they hear you say their child needs to be assessed. Many argue with you and deny it. It's easier to talk if you know the families and they trust you. When children change caregivers frequently, it can be overwhelming for caregivers, and the parents are overwhelmed too. It's easier to work on problems when you've been with parents for a while and you're comfortable with each other.

The mother of a young child diagnosed with obsessive-compulsive disorder thinks her son's caregiver is more responsive and caring because she knows him so well. She explains,

> High-maintenance children like my son take a lot of patience. You have to like a child to treat him well, and not all children are easy to like. Consistency of care has reduced [my son's] stress level and made him easier to care for. The caregiver knows how to treat him and what to expect. He does much better under these conditions.

For families. Continuity over time has clear benefits for parents as well as children. As the caregiver-child bond grows stronger, parents are relieved, reassured, and ultimately grateful for the caregiver's place in their lives. They can go to work knowing that their child is in the arms of someone who cares deeply about him. One mother notes,

What I like best is the relationship with the caregiver. I know her, and she knows me and Aaron. I know the relationship will last a long time—until we're ready for the change to preschool. In that way it's like family child care. I don't have to keep getting used to new caregivers and neither does my son.

Continuity gives caregivers the groundwork they need to help families navigate life's changes. A child's grandmother gets sick and needs long-term medical care; a new baby sister is born; a single parent invites her sister and her children to move in until they can find a place of their own. Caregivers in relationships with parents over time can see a child's behavior contextually, so they are prepared to help both the child and the parents weather change and crisis with insight, grace, and humor. Explains one such caregiver,

> The child can be herself in the child care setting—and doesn't have to do or be what adults ask of her [elsewhere]. She doesn't have to sit quietly or wait when adults have problems to solve or too much to do. Continuity gives children something they count on when they are away from their parents and home life. For children at risk, it may be all they have to count on.

A parent appreciative of the policy adds, "When a family has troubles, the child has an adult to count on—someone who'll be waiting for her every day. She knows that part of her life is settled, predictable."

When a center practices continuity of care, every adult knows the care relationship will last for several years, so they work to build trust and understanding. Parents know they will be heard if they make suggestions, and they assume the caregiver will ask them for advice if she needs it. They feel it is worth the time to share information about their child's sleep patterns, interactions with siblings, food preferences, and relationships with grandparents.

When there are differences, families and caregivers work harder because they know the relationship is there to stay. One teacher admits,

> I've had trouble getting along with a few parents. Usually it was because we had different styles or philosophies. In one case the mother wasn't good at reading her child's cues. She would overstimulate him so that by the time he arrived at the center, he would be hyper. After she left, I would have to figure out a way to calm him down. It was frustrating, but I worked hard to get along with the mom because I knew the relationship wasn't going away.

Long-term, continuous relationships enable parents and caregivers to define childrearing goals and values at a natural pace. Parents take

"Continuity gives children something they count on when they are away from their parents and home life."

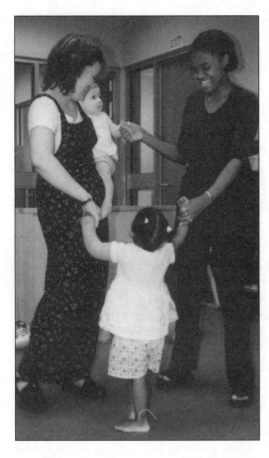

risks, sharing their views on bottle feeding, nursing, and responding to babies who fuss. Caregivers become open to learning how parents discipline. What rules do they set? What are the consequences if rules are not followed? This process is strengthened as parents see the child-caregiver bond grow.

The value parents place on their relationship with a caregiver is evident when families plan pregnancies so the baby will be born when their favorite caregiving team is ready to return to the infant room. Some mothers and fathers in the University of New Mexico's program have gone so far as to ask to have their not-yet-conceived babies placed on the center's waiting list!

For caregivers. Every caregiver we interviewed who offers continuity of care credits that policy for deepening her understanding of family circumstances. Some also attribute their success, at least in part, to the age at which the children enter the program, supporting the view that the earlier a child enters care, the more important the continuity of relationships. One teacher notes,

> It is easier to form relationships with parents when children are very young. . . . Parents go out of their way to get to know us and build teamwork. When children are older, parents are less interested in a relationship with their child's caregiver. They think children should be able to handle the separation because they've done it many times already.

One thoughtful caregiver explains that continuity of care makes it easier for her to manage the inevitable conflicts with families:

> I was worried that I'd be stuck for three years with a group of parents I didn't like. But as I learned more I began to think of working through tensions or conflicts with the parent as a professional challenge rather than a source of stress. The benefits of this kind of care began to outweigh the negatives.

Her coworker agrees:

> I think parents work harder at developing relationships with us now because they know the relationships will last over time. Parents aren't inclined to develop close relationships when they know the child will be moving soon.

Relationships, the Heart of Quality Care

Low pay and few benefits undoubtedly contribute to child care's high staff turnover, but continuity of care can positively influence caregiver job satisfaction and a caregiver's willingness to stay in a program. One teacher, on the same caregiving team for four years, says of her coworker,

> We've been together long enough to read each other's body language. I can tell when she's stressed and needs help, and she can tell the same about me. We've developed the same philosophy and the same style. I've learned a lot from watching her, and she says she's learned from me. I really enjoy our teamwork.

For directors and centers. We began our research believing that continuity of care is a valuable strategy that raises the level of quality by encouraging warm, responsive, long-term relationships between staff and families. What we were not prepared for was the overwhelming enthusiasm of every staff member and every parent involved. When we asked directors how their staff accept moving with the children each year and how parents feel about it, the common reply was, "They *love* it!" Better care, a happy staff, strong relationships, and less turnover: What more could a director or center want from a child care policy?

"I think parents work harder at developing relationships with us now because they know the relationships will last over time."

Moving toward continuity of care

When people understand child development, the concept of continuity of care makes sense. The barriers to implementation are most often logistical rather than philosophical. How can programs change staff attitudes when caregivers are resistant? How do they manage staffing patterns? How can centers meet state staffing ratios and still balance their budgets? How do programs go about making the transition to full continuity of care? Let's look at one program as a case study.

When the University of New Mexico (UNM) child care center began taking a serious look at continuity of care, the youngest child in its program was 12 months old. Says the program's current director,

> When we began, we weren't sure babies should be in group care, because we weren't sure we could meet their needs. To make up our minds, we started reading everything we could find on attachment and met together to discuss what we had read. We wanted to know what brain research said about child development. What was special or different about infant/ toddler care?

The UNM staff also sought out experts. Together, they explored the research and philosophy underlying the approach, especially with babies. They observed a program in Houston that offered continuity of care and talked with Ron Lally, codirector of the Center for Child & Family Studies at WestEd, a nonprofit research, development, and service agency. Janet Gonzalez-Mena, who writes about multicultural issues, helped them think about supporting cultural differences. Internationally recognized leader in infant care Magda Gerber helped them envision environments of patient and respectful staff supporting babies' exploration and growth. The center also spent time discussing the logistics of the transition. Which caregiving team would go to the baby room for the first infant/toddler rotation? At the end of each year, would the children change rooms or remain where they were? How would the staff explain continuity of care to families? A two-day retreat helped them work through such questions.

> One of our concerns had to do with primary caregiving. We wanted to be sure both adults [on the caregiving team] knew as much as possible about all of the children. . . . We didn't want to put a stress on the child if one of the adults was gone. We didn't want the infant room to turn into two tiny classrooms where either caregiver might say, "I'll get your teacher to change your diaper."

It took nine months of research before the UNM staff decided to care for infants. In August 1996 three teachers volunteered for the new assignment. But even after the center opened to babies, staff learning continued. They used a curriculum called *Keys to Caregiving* (Barnard & Sumner 1996), from the University of Washington in Seattle. Workshops for caregivers and parents were held on caregiver-child attachments, preparing for babies, being with babies in the second year, and separation. Still there were glitches.

> We had to work through problems even after the program was up and running. It was too expensive for us to fully equip all three rooms [for the entire age range], so we planned that the caregivers and children would change rooms each year. We agreed that the caregiving team . . . could arrange and decorate the new room any way they wanted when they moved in. This turned out to be hard. The first set of caregivers had made the room comfy for themselves, and then the new team came along and rearranged it. The first team felt hurt. They had to remember that children coming in are younger than the children who are leaving. But we found that changing rooms had benefits because it showed the caregivers how much the children had grown. In the new room with new equipment they discovered the new things their children could do.

In January 2003, after three infant/toddler rotations, the center decided to enroll babies into the program in January as well as September. "We were missing a lot of summer babies," explains the director. "They had to be 6 weeks by September 15 to enter the program. Families had to wait a year if their children were born after July 6. Now those children can enter in January." The director doesn't know how they'll manage when the children are ready to move to preschool. "We're hoping there'll be openings. If there aren't, we'll just have to figure out what to do. But that's what we've been doing all along." The staff at the UNM child care center are still learning. (For more about this program, see **Two Continuity of Care Exemplars.**)

Even when programs recognize that continuity of care is good, especially for very young children, their families, and caregivers, they may feel overwhelmed by the challenges that come with implementation. Continuity of care affects staffing, use of rooms and space, finances, attitudes, hiring, and organization of the whole center. Directors worry: "How can I convince my toddler teacher—the best one I've ever had—to work with babies?" "My infant room is too small to fit toddlers; will I have to renovate the building?" "How can I balance my budget if I have to re-staff all the rooms at the ratio set for babies?"

Two Continuity of Care Exemplars

The **University of New Mexico Children's Campus for Early Care and Education** and **Grossmont College Child Care** both have well-established infant/toddler programs that offer continuity of care.

The staff in both centers are skilled at developing warm relationships with children birth to age 3 in mixed-age groupings. They know how to manage children's transition into care and know what to do to help parents and children reduce separation anxiety. They are skilled at reading babies' cues and understand differences in personality and temperament. They value toddlers' bids for independence and know how to support diverse childrearing styles and priorities.

Grossmont College, near San Diego, is the demonstration site in Southern California for WestEd's Program for Infant/Toddler Caregivers (PITC) Partners for Quality. WestEd's Center for Child & Family Studies works with the California Department of Education to increase the supply and quality of infant/toddler child care and dev- elopment services in the state. The program recruits and trains new and experienced center-based caregivers and family child care providers; develops infrastructures at the local and regional levels to increase the supply and quality of services for children from birth through age 3; and supports an infrastructure that provides training and technical assistance for infant/toddler caregivers.

PITC has developed a wealth of educational materials and videos to support its goals. Its demonstration programs operate at six community college campuses (including Grossmont) in five regions of California, where students, directors, policy makers, and other visitors can observe the PITC philosophy of infant/toddler care in action. For more information about PITC, visit www.pitc.org.

The section that follows explores these problems and some of the solutions successful programs have used in making the transition to continuity of care.

Fiscal barriers. The money challenge is one of the biggest hurdles to continuity of care. For the most part, the barrier has to do with the higher labor costs of infant care. Because of staff-child ratio requirements, it's much more expensive to care for infants and toddlers when they share the same room than it is to care for them separately. If, for example, state regulations require staff-child ratios of 1:4 for infants and 1:6 for toddlers, a center with broad age groupings and mixed ages of 6 weeks to 18 months would have to staff the room at the lower ratio. Directors ask: "How can we overcome the ratio issue and remain fiscally healthy?" Some end the discussion there. But there are ways to overcome fiscal challenges. Here are six to consider.

■ *Create a sliding fee scale*

Realizing that instability was a problem for children in its care, the U.S. Army introduced a system of continuity of care that offers food for thought. According to the chief of child development programs, Headquarters, U.S. Army,

> Previously, the Army used ratios as the guideline for moving children [when there were openings or slots to fill]. . . . [But] when we mapped out children's moves and the turnover rate and the times that parents [relocate] or are deployed, we realized that what we were doing wasn't good for children. In the military, sometimes the caregiver is the most stable person in a child's life.

Developers decided that rather than cluster children narrowly by age, the first grouping would include children birth to 18 months old. Infants and toddlers could remain with a caregiving team until they were 40 months old; staff-child ratios do not exceed recommended group size for the age of the child. The Army's next challenge was to find a way to share the financial burden. It solved this problem by basing its rates on the parents' ability to pay.

> People who have [infants as opposed to older children] are the least likely to be able to afford child care. In our case, that's Privates. Privates don't make a lot of money, and so [we decided they would] pay less for care.

The Army's approach reverses the standard practice of charging parents of infants the highest fee. Its policy makers stressed the priority of offering children quality care from the beginning, and the fee structure followed.

Directors ask: "How can we overcome the ratio issue and remain fiscally healthy?"

■ *Offer scholarships*

Not all centers can offer a sliding fee scale. In New York, for example, programs providing care that is subsidized by the state aren't permitted to charge less to parents who pay tuition out of their own pockets. Child care programs that serve a mix of public and privately funded children struggle with this fee structure—especially when some parents' yearly earnings are only a few hundred dollars over the cutoff for public assistance. A director explains,

> We can't set a lower rate for private-pay families. Instead, we help parents [who must pay with personal funds] and can't afford full fees by creating a scholarship line in our budget. In effect, we set aside a portion of our income to subsidize private pay families. The County doesn't object as long as our budget shows how we generate the money. We determine the total cost of care and give small scholarships to parents who lack the means to pay the full price.

It's difficult to offer scholarships when you're operating on a tight budget, but it's better than leaving an opening unfilled. Says a director,

> The way I look at it, half an income is better than no income at all. If you have to pay for two people to staff a room for eight children and you only have six or seven children, why not take one more on scholarship. Sure, your income is less than it would be if the person paid full price; but it will cover your increased cost for food and supplies. Your fixed costs don't change, so you're still ahead. At the same time, you have to be careful not to give away so many scholarships that you damage your whole program. You don't want say "I'm child care, so I can get by with less."

For this director, a limited number of scholarships is a way of maximizing revenue.

■ *Charge a flat rate*

Creativity is another important tool for balancing income with expenses. Some programs charge all families the same rate, regardless of the age of the child. This approach lifts the burden from parents of infants and toddlers, spreading the cost of care across all the families who use the center. It also relieves administrative staff responsible for record keeping. At the Miami Dade College–Wolfson Campus Child Development Center, an administrator says, "It used to be a bookkeeping nightmare when we set fees based on income or the number of credits a student was taking in school. The flat rate is much easier." The comparison in **Cost-of-Care Rate vs. Flat Rate** (on page 112) shows surprising little difference between an age-varied rate and a flat rate, making the latter an option worth exploring.

Cost-of-Care Rate vs. Flat Rate

For the same number of children, the same income can result by adjusting the fee schedule.

Hypothetical using cost-of-care rate

8 infants @ $150/week = $1,200

16 toddlers @ $135/week = $2,160

50 preschoolers @ $130/week = $6,500

Total income/week = $9,860

Hypothetical using flat rate

74 children @ $130/week, regardless of age

Total income/week = $9,620

■ *Secure in-kind support*

Some programs cover the cost of care by working out financial arrangements with a convenient campus or business. Programs might negotiate support for space, overhead, maintenance, advertising, and billing from the campus or corporation in return for slots for its students or employees/clients. The degree to which a large organization supports a child care program is dependent on good politics and plenty of relationship building.

■ *Look at the budget overall*

Regional trainers/coordinators for WestEd's Program for Infant/Toddler Caregivers (PITC) suggest that directors let other parts of their program support infant/toddler care:

> Some centers with strong preschool programs may want to use the infant program as a feeder program to preschool. Say, for example, there are 16 infants and toddlers and 100 preschoolers. The director will want to look at the break-even point. She'll spread out the dollars so the preschool program helps cover the cost of the infant/toddler program. The infant/toddler families will become the core, because the children will stay through preschool. Families will spread the word, and the program will grow.

At the University of Michigan Health Systems Child Care Center, a summer school-age program helps support infant/toddler care:

> A lot of these [older] children went through our infant/toddler and preschool programs and now they go to different schools. They return to the summer camp because the relationships formed in our early programs were so strong. Families come at 5:00 in the morning on registration day and stand in line to enroll their children.

■ *Help parents re-value the benefits of continuity*

In some centers the only solution is to raise fees to cover the higher costs of quality care. But it isn't easy for a center to change its fee structure, especially when parents are used to paying less. The Wolfson Center, for example, decided to establish continuity of care first.

> We wanted parents to experience the benefits of the program so that they knew what they were paying for. We told parents, "We aren't out to make money; we're just trying to pay for high-quality care." The parents accepted the change because they could see the difference in the program.

Given enough information, parents with sufficient resources are usually willing to pay more for the benefits of continuity of care.

Centers that look to the corporate world for ideas and advice on how to stay solvent often implement policies and practices focused on efficiency, large groupings, assembly-line care. They focus on costs, downplaying children's need for attachment and relationship in order to keep expenses low. However, even some sectors of corporate America recognize that low prices are not the only way, or necessarily the best way, to keep customers happy. Instead, they are discovering the high value their customers place on individualized attention, flexibility, trust, collaboration, personal loyalty. In other words, business is finding out what relationship-focused centers already know: the "secret to success" is *relationships.* Once centers acknowledge individualized care and community as their priority, the added costs of relationship-based care becomes easier to "sell" to parents.

Regulatory obstacles. Some states have regulations that prohibit centers from mixing children younger than 18 months (or 2 years) old with children who are older. Directors who see the advantages of continuity of care are naturally frustrated. Says one, "Our babies become attached to their caregivers, but according to state regulations, we have to move children along when they turn 18 months." And another, "A child enters the toddler room at 14 months and then when she turns 2—after 10 months of bonding with her original caregiver—our state regs say she has to move up."

It may seem that a director's hands are tied in such states, but this isn't necessarily so; states can waive their regulations, depending on circumstances. In New York, for example, if the center's goal is to provide high-quality care and the program has a good track record, the state will make an exception. New Mexico's Children, Youth, and Families Department gave the UNM child care center a waiver to mix children under and over 2 years of age. On the application, the director emphasized that the program was unique, and she outlined the rotation system:

Given enough information, parents with sufficient resources are usually willing to pay more for the benefits of continuity of care.

Example of Continuity Rotations

Members of a caregiver team are kept together unless someone leaves or is promoted.

	Year 1	Year 2	Year 3	Year 4	Year 5	Year 6
Team #1	New group of young infants enter the program (in the Infant Room)	Team #1 and children stay together, but in a new room	Team #1 and children stay together, but in a new room	*Children go to preschool* *Team #1 starts over with a new group of young infants in the Infant Room*		
Team #2		New group of young infants enter the program (in the Infant Room)	Team #2 and children stay together, but in a new room	Team #2 and children stay together, but in a new room	*Children go to preschool* *Team #2 starts over with a new group of young infants in the Infant Room*	
Team #3			New group of young infants enter the program (in the Infant Room)	Team #3 and children stay together, but in a new room	Team #3 and children stay together, but in a new room	*Children go to preschool* *Team #3 starts over with a new group of young infants in the Infant Room*

We explained that there would be some overlap in ages in the toddler room. . . . The state wants what's best for children too. New Mexico is on the low end for staff-child ratios and quality care. But you can get waivers for innovative programs. You have to get to know the licensing folks. We got into a dialogue with them and built a relationship, and so the waiver was possible.

Other states may also consider waivers. The key lies in making the case that the change will improve the quality of care for children.

Staffing logistics. Continuity of care is often intimidating because it can entail changing the staffing pattern of the whole center. Says one director,

Relationships, the Heart of Quality Care

Example of Continuity Rotations, in a Program That Can't Mix Children under and over 18 Months

Children move with their primary caregiver until they go on to preschool, then the adult loops back to begin again with a younger group.

Year 1	Year 2	Year 3	Year 4
Infant Room One caregiver (Bertha) is assigned to the four youngest children One caregiver (Abby) is assigned to the four oldest children	**Mobile Infant Room #1** Four youngest children from the Infant Room and their primary caregiver (Bertha) Plus four new children from the waiting list and a second primary caregiver (Harry) **Mobile Infant Room #2 (Pretoddler)** Four oldest children from the Infant Room and their primary caregiver (Abby) Plus four new children from the waiting list and a second primary caregiver (Gail)	**Toddler Room #1** All eight children and both caregivers (Bertha, Harry) move together from Mobile Infant Room #1 **Toddler Room #2 (Older)** All eight children and both caregivers (Abby, Gail) move together from Mobile Infant Room #2	*All children in Toddler Rooms #1 and #2 move to preschool* *All caregivers move back: Abby and Bertha to the Infant Room and Gail and Harry to a Mobile Infant Room (Gail to #1, Harry to #2) each to be paired with a different caregiver moving up from the Infant Room this time*

I'd like to implement continuity of care, but I just can't figure out how to do it. Do the children stay in the same room or do they change rooms at the end of the year? Do I move the children one by one or as a group to preschool? What do I do with children who enroll mid-year? It's just too complicated!

Centers resolve these questions in several different ways. At the Miami-Dade College–Wolfson Campus Child Development Center, each September a group of children aged 6 weeks to 11 months enters the program and is assigned a team of teachers and given a name (e.g., "Butterflies"). The following September, when the Butterflies are 12–23 months old, they and their caregivers change rooms together. A new group of young infants aged 6 weeks to 11 months enters, is assigned caregivers, and gets a name (e.g., "Sunflowers"). The next September, when the Butterflies are 24–35 months old and the Sunflowers are 12–23 months old, the groups and their caregivers again move; and a third group of young infants enters (e.g., "Teddy Bears"). A year after that, the Butterflies, now 36–47 months old, depart for preschool together, freeing their caregivers to begin with a new group of children, and a new rotation. The Sunflowers and Teddy Bears each move up one room as well. Each room at the center contains materials matched to the developmental abilities of children of that age. This kind of rotation is captured in the figure **Example of Continuity Rotations** (on page 114).

"If I have a new teacher, I can pair her with a seasoned caregiver who can act as her mentor."

Because the Wolfson Campus program has two rooms for children aged 12–23 months and two rooms for children aged 24–35 months, each September it is also able to form a new group of children who are enrolling for the first time at 12–23 months old (e.g., "Bluebirds"). Depending on their ages, newly enrolling children may also join one of the existing groups (Butterflies, Sunflowers, Teddy Bears), if openings exist. When a group goes off to preschool and its caregiver team starts over, the team may be assigned either to the next 6 weeks–11 month group or to the next 12–23 month group.

In states that don't permit centers to mix children under 18 months with older children, staffing logistics are more complicated, but continuity is still an option. In one such center, the infant room houses eight children birth to 9 months and two caregivers. At the end of the year the eight children are separated: One of the caregivers goes with the four youngest children to the mobile infant room, and the other caregiver goes with the four oldest to the pretoddler room. Four new children from the waiting list are added in each room, along with a second caregiver. The next year, the caregivers and children move up together to the two toddler rooms. The year after that all 16 children move on to preschool, and the four caregivers return to assignments with younger groups. **Example of Continuity Rotations, in a Program That Can't Mix Children under and over 18 Months** (on page 115) shows such a progression.

In this continuity model the caregiving teams can be fluid. A director who follows this model explains:

> We have 10 infant/toddler teachers and five rooms. We don't try to keep caregiving teams together throughout the whole three-year rotation, but we do keep the children with at least one of the caregivers. All 10

Relationships, the Heart of Quality Care

caregivers understand that they aren't the focus; their job is to meet the needs of the children.

She adds that she likes the flexibility of such a system:

> If I have a new teacher, I can pair her with a seasoned caregiver who can act as her mentor. The system is also good for breaking up cliques. It stops teachers from saying, "I don't want to work with her." The teachers know they all have to work together. I'm able to place teachers where they are strongest or put them with coworkers who have strengths that are complementary.

Staffing a center with teachers who are committed, or at least open, to a system of continuity makes rotation logistics even easier to deal with. This is the strategy taken by the Gallup Organization Child Development Center (CDC) in Lincoln, Nebraska, an employer-owned program licensed to serve 150 children. The center organizes the younger children into small "family" groups of one caregiver and three to five infants. As the group ages, children on the waiting list are added, raising the number to five to seven toddlers. Children stay with their family group and their caregiver until they turn 3. Some teachers have even moved with their family groups to the center's preschool. The value that CDC places on attachment through continuity is reflected in its employment procedures.

> CDC hires teachers with a style that favors forming relationships, using as a resource the ECTP, or Early Childhood Teacher Perceiver (SRI 1989). The ECTP is a structured interview that takes about 25 minutes to complete. A profile results, showing each teacher-candidate's configuration on 10 key themes. These themes include relationship qualities, such as empathy and rapport. . . . Because the program philosophy requires continuity, CDC asks new as well as renewing teachers to commit [to stay] the two to three years it takes children [in their "family"] to reach age 3. (Raikes 1996, 64)

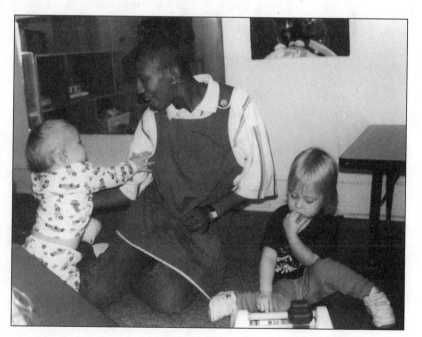

At the end of each rotation, CDC's caregivers

are encouraged to re-evaluate their career goals and determine their readiness to commit to another family group.

Space for mixed-age groups. In the last decade many child care centers built small, cozy infant rooms designed for a few nonmobile babies, cribs, high chairs, a changing table, and a quiet place for napping. Such a space is ideal for rocking and carrying babies who are too young to walk, but children had to move on when they became mobile. Centers that want to offer a relationship-based program and continuity of care have to look at that space differently. Some renovate their buildings so they can care for infants and toddlers in the same room. Others increase their useable indoor space by permitting toddlers to sleep on mats that can be stacked rather than in separate nap rooms.

Once ages are mixed, a different kind of supervision and attention is required from adults. Toddlers who are unsteady on their feet can trip over babies on blankets or hug the babies too tight or kiss them too hard. One teacher says, "We worry that the babies will be hurt by the toddlers, and parents worry about that too. It's harder to ensure the safety of children when you mix age groups."

Nothing replaces good, old-fashioned adult attentiveness, but there are as many ingenious ways to address the problem of mixing infants and toddlers as there are safety-minded caregivers. Some put nonmobile infants in swings or umbrella strollers, even backpacks, to keep them out of toddler reach. High-sided fabric "nests," pillows, or pillow pits; plastic wading pools without water; and out-of-the-way blanket areas can keep babies safe from older children on the move. Low, carpeted platforms, surrounded by clear panels and designed with safety in mind, can permit maximum mobility while keeping babies out of danger from toddlers' newly dancing feet. Portable logs or dividers, which create boundaries and divide the room, are also helpful. So are indoor climbers, if the equipment is used conscientiously. (For more on safety, see Greenman 1988.) A teacher explains,

> We use toddler climbing equipment to help control the flow of movement and activity. The toddlers love it because they like to climb and step up, and we like it because it removes them from the babies. We also look at the flow of activity between the indoors and the outdoors. When the weather is warm, the [younger and older] children can be kept farther apart.

There is no question that mixed-age groupings require more adult attention, or at least attention of a different kind. But it's also the case that the small groups and primary caregiving typical of continuity of

Relationships, the Heart of Quality Care

care make it easier for caregivers to focus on each child as an individual—easier, perhaps, than trying to attend to the needs of a classroom full of same-age children. As in a loving family, toddlers in a mixed-age group are often more of a help than a hindrance. They learn to nurture babies as part of their own special care group. Reports one previously resistant caregiver,

> All it took for me to become convinced of the advantages of continuity of care was to observe one of my toddlers lovingly patting his 4-month-old friend to sleep. I began to imagine that baby, six months down the road, laughing with delight as she tries to follow her more mobile classmates on a romp through the room. When I got to the part in my fantasy where I see the two of them, like a little family, growing up with me over several years, I was sold.

Negative attitudes. Overcoming structural barriers such as finances and staffing is hard enough, but sometimes changes "just don't feel right." Here are two objections that some directors, teachers, and parents often make to continuity of care.

■ *"My toddler teacher doesn't want to care for babies"*

Despite its advantages, many caregivers who are used to working in programs with traditional groupings resist the idea of continuity of care. Some caregivers find toddlers lively and delightful and are proud of their ability to work with an age group that tries the patience of others. They may threaten to quit if they have to care for babies too. Caregivers in the infant room can be equally vocal about caring for anyone *but* babies. Centers that get such a response may decide to defer to caregiver preferences and leave policies unchanged in order to keep reliable workers in a field already plagued by high staff turnover.

Regional trainers/coordinators from PITC Partners for Quality work hard to help centers overcome such attitudes. The effort has to start with the director.

> The directors have to pass the vision on to the staff. They have to think of the larger vision—the whole program for children birth to 3. They can't think classroom by classroom. Directors have to be willing to sacrifice the individual caregiver for the whole center. When they post ads for new staff, they should state that they are looking for people who are willing to care for infants *and* toddlers. During the interview, they should tell prospective employees that they may be asked to move along with the children. Little by little, directors will begin to replace [resistant] staff with people who understand the ideal and are prepared to make it happen.

There are other approaches besides *all or nothing*. PITC has this suggestion:

As a first step, directors can reduce the number of times children change caregivers. They can move babies once a year, instead of twice, and make sure that at least one familiar caregiver remains with the group. At the same time, they can make sure that everyone on staff receives intensive training [on caring for young children at various ages].

In many excellent centers, continuity is encouraged and valued but not insisted on for each caregiver. Some teachers move with the children, while others stay with their preferred age group. These centers pull from the best of both worlds. Some caregivers become skilled with one particular age or stage, and some become adept at long-term relationships with children and adults. By working together they learn from each other, and everyone benefits.

■ *"But parents want their children to move every year!"*

Some parents carry memories of their school days into the early care setting. Each fall they expect their children to change teachers and "pass" to the next "grade." Programs or parents who resist continuity of care because families would miss "moving up" act to children's detriment. Says one frustrated director, "At our center we haven't been able to discontinue these annual parties. Parents look forward to their children's 'graduations' all year long. These small ceremonies give parents a chance to celebrate the milestones in their children's lives."

But there is no need to stop the parties, just the yearly changes. Once they are helped to understand the value of continuity of care and

---

Ten Tips for Centers Making the Transition to Continuity of Care

1. Reflect together on children's development with and without continuity.

2. Sort out the pros and cons of primary caregiving as a practice.

3. Make transition plans together; think about including families too.

4. Hire and train caregivers to work with children birth to 3.

5. Hire and train caregivers to work in multi-age settings.

6. Educate caregivers to focus on the whole child, not just on the age of the child.

7. Build teamwork among staff; partner expert infant caregivers with expert toddler caregivers to build staff competencies informally.

8. Hire caregivers who are willing to stay with the same children for more than one year.

9. As an interim step toward full continuity, let one caregiver move up with the children and keep one "expert" caregiver behind to greet the new group and maintain center-wide continuity.

10. Educate families about the importance of continuity; share testimonies from parents and caregivers who have experience with it.

Relationships, the Heart of Quality Care

primary caregiving, families can learn to celebrate the caregiver-child relationship rather than the "graduations" that divide children from the adults they have come to trust and love.

> When my first child was ready to make the change to the toddler room, I came to the center and celebrated her "graduation." The children looked so cute and we all had cookies, like a real party. However, the next day my daughter cried and cried because she couldn't be with Lisa [her infant caregiver]. The new caregiver wasn't the same. I told her she was a big girl now, but she was devastated every time we walked past Lisa's door.

There are better ways to acknowledge growth in children. Strong parent-caregiver ties make the absence of "graduations" easier, because families come to trust the center's lead. Attachment becomes the best celebration of all.

Becoming committed to continuity of care is the first and biggest step toward bringing the idea into form. **Ten Tips for Centers Making the Transition to Continuity of Care** offers some guidance.

Strategy #4: Smooth transitions

All sorts of transitions have to be navigated by young children in group care—beginning and ending relationships, moving from lunch to naps, clean-up time, going outside and coming back in again, to name just a few. Some children adapt to new things more easily than others. Some go with the flow no matter what; others need help day-to-day; and still others need structure, predictability, and a sensitive caregiver to make even small disruptions, like diaper changes or washing up for lunch, go smoothly. Transitions can prompt tantrums and tears, challenging behavior, or withdrawal. Whether children are easy-going, sensitive, or tightly wound, all benefit from smooth routines and time to adjust to changes in their lives.

Good directors and caregivers are well positioned to plan constructive transitions. Directors especially set the tone, by orchestrating timing and communication. They know that ignoring a child's feelings during a transition hampers adjustment and prolongs grief. Here is the story of one kindergarten teacher who learned to appreciate the importance of well-planned transitions, no matter what the child's age:

> Antonio cried every single morning when his mother left for work. He would go up to the book loft and sob for almost an hour. He didn't want any attention or consolation; he just wanted to grieve alone, privately. I had never seen a 5-year-old have such a hard time adjusting.

After the first month I scheduled a conference with his mother and learned that this was Antonio's first time away from home. She had been an at-home mom, and he was her last baby. Neither of us had understood that he needed more preparation than children who had simply moved up from the 4-year-old room. We were both surprised at how long his transition was taking, but she was sure he would be okay—she knew him as a bright and resilient child. We agreed to watch and wait and talk with him about his feelings, as much as he would allow.

With our combined support Antonio slowly began to join activities and even occasionally would smile and forget himself in our classroom fun. By December he only went up to the book loft out of habit, and usually ended up coming right back down to play with the other children. By January he was the happiest, most intelligent, and creative child I have ever worked with.

Benefits of smooth transitions

For children. Well-planned transitions allow a child to see life as stable and predictable. They minimize disruption and keep children's needs a priority. Smooth transitions recognize and respect the deep attachments children have formed with beloved caregivers, and they teach children life lessons about dealing with separation and loss.

For families. Families also benefit from well-orchestrated transition routines and adequate adjustment time. Until their special caregiver is no longer around, many parents do not recognize the important place she has held in their children's lives and in their own. Smooth, thoughtful, professionally handled transitions give parents time to navigate challenges and deal with everyone's inevitable feelings of loss.

For caregivers. Constructive transition routines can be empowering. Caregivers feel professional and proud of navigating yet another adjustment process and preparing for a new group of families. Transitions give caregivers a sense of closure that is useful in managing a job full of bonded relationships. Planned changes maintain clear and healthy boundaries that define the caregiver's role as a temporary substitute for parents. And finally, when transitions are predictable and orderly, children negotiate them more effectively—and that makes it easier for everyone.

For directors and centers. We have seen a direct connection between transitions and turnover. Families as well as caregivers are more likely to change centers when bonds are frequently disrupted and life feels unstable, sad, or chaotic. When transitions are smooth,

"We agreed to watch and wait and talk with him about his feelings, as much as he would allow."

the adults are more likely to stay put—and that means centers can continue to offer quality care even while change is in progress.

Moving toward smooth transitions

Experienced caregivers, who have been through transitions many times with many families, develop coping mechanisms for dealing with the loss of daily contact with the children and adults they care about. Experienced caregivers share what they know to help everyone manage the passages.

Ensure that first transitions are positive. A child's first transition—his beginning in child care—can be the most important. Whether children begin child care as infants or are older (like Antonio), they need to be eased into their new situations with sensitivity and thoughtfulness. Lessons learned from the University of New Mexico child care center are useful for children of any age. In that relationship-based model, newly enrolling parents of children up to age 2½ must agree to spend at least a week helping their child adjust to the new arrangement. At first parents go a short distance, to a small room just outside the classroom door. If children become upset, parents return to comfort and soothe. Gradually they leave the center for longer periods of time.

The transition takes place at the child's pace. Children are helped to understand that parents leave and parents come back, and that coming and going is natural. By the time a parent stays away a full day, the child has realized that important people come back, even if it takes some time. The idea is to relieve child and parent of the stress of separation and to strengthen the parent-caregiver-child triad. Ideally, by the end of the transition period children are comfortable and parents feel they can trust the caregiver to act on their behalf.

A slowly evolved transition such as the one at UNM gives caregivers and parents a chance to observe each other's interactions with the children, which in turn clues them in to expectations and routines at home and at the center. With parents nearby and children relaxed and content, caregivers have an opportunity to begin learning each child's unique temperament, preferences, and cues. A caregiver sees whether a new baby likes to rock or finger a blanket when he goes to sleep. A father might discover his child likes being carried in a Snuggli as much as sitting and looking around in an infant seat. A teacher can see how a mother deals with a child who startles easily or how a grandmother offers food. Having a chance to listen to families'

Children are helped to understand that parents leave and parents come back, and that coming and going is natural.

words and note their small interactions can be of great help to caregivers when parents are no longer around.

Plan orderly changes. Centers that deal thoughtfully and effectively with transitions tend to move children in predictable patterns, keep them with familiar peers and caregivers as much as possible, and allow plenty of time for everyone to adjust. When a change in rooms is coming, children are offered several weeks—even a month—of progressively longer daily visits to their new classrooms. Teachers help them ease into new routines and friendships. Many children move up with their friends.

The current and future caregivers usually orchestrate the transition between old and new classrooms. Once the move is complete, children might be allowed to visit old classrooms or find former caregivers on the playground. Typically, children and families manage planned transitions admirably and settle in with minimal disruption. Matter-of-fact attitudes and approaches help children and families adjust with increasing ease to regular changes, which are an accepted and expected part of American child care center life today.

Keep the process constructive. Whether transitions are frequent or rare, disruption and to some extent grief are always a part of the

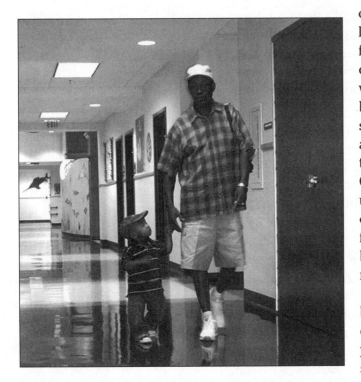

equation and must be taken into consideration in each transition plan. In best practice, children are not faulted for having trouble with changes or for needing to touch base with former caregivers. Challenging behaviors, withdrawal, clinginess, sadness, anger, and abrupt swings in attachment are understood as part of the process and taken in stride. Children are given the extra time and understanding they need to create closure with beloved caregivers, friends, and familiar routines before being moved forward into new relationships.

Some caregivers make scrapbooks and memory folders for children and families to revisit over the years. They understand that keepsakes and rituals such as these help everyone to deal with grief and to let go constructively. There are also good-bye parties, "graduations," and other commonly used transition tools. Families sometimes honor caregivers with mementos. In the best of situations, centers allow post-transition visiting and keep boundaries between children and beloved caregivers flexible and loose. Families are encouraged to be involved every step of the way.

Help adults transition too. Children aren't the only ones who need help with transitions. At the UNM child care center, which offers continuity of care for infants and toddlers, staff were taken by surprise when the first group of children made their transition to the preschool classroom. Parents had a hard time letting go of their relationships with the infant/toddler team and were slow to develop new relationships with their children's new preschool teachers.

The preschool staff knew that this difference in closeness was partly developmental. Caregivers don't need to touch base with parents as often once children become more independent. But something else was at work too. The parents were missing the easy give-and-take that had been part of their close relationships with the infant/toddler teachers, so they continued to seek out their children's first caregivers when they had questions or needed reassurance. The parents weren't moving on.

The infant/toddler staff realized that in future transitions they had to help families change their focus, to detach constructively from old, treasured relationships and make room for new ones. To this end, the infant/toddler team began talking with parents about what to expect in preschool. They helped parents understand that infant/toddler caregivers usually nurture children and their families on a deep level; and that preschool caregivers offer support too, but from a greater distance. Developmentally, children under 3 rely almost totally on adults to anticipate their needs. But 3- and 4-year-olds, with their growing sense of independence and accomplishment, crave respect and autonomy; they can talk about their day and articulate their needs for themselves. This developmental difference makes parents and caregivers somewhat less important as sources of information, because children can serve in that role. Relationships between the adults in the preschool are less intense.

At the same time, the preschool teachers in this program decided to become more proactive. They gave family tours, hosted potluck dinners and parties for transitioning parents, and wrote a booklet describing their program. Parents appreciated these gestures and made suggestions of their own. When we last visited the center, the

Constructive transitions can take many forms, but the need for thoughtful planning can never be overrated or dismissed.

preschool transition was smoother and relationships were thriving in both settings.

A proactive approach is also helpful when children leave the center for another institution. In the best of cases, center staff work with families and new schools in ways similar to those described above. Careful planning can make this important change as manageable as ones navigated earlier. It certainly can prevent situations like this one described by a caregiver.

> Serena was a bright and articulate 6-year-old who taught herself to read and do simple addition during kindergarten. Near the end of the year, without alerting us, her mom brought her to a local prep school to take an entrance test. Serena consciously and determinedly blew the test! On the way home she proudly announced, "I didn't tell them the answers."

Strategies for Orchestrating Smooth Transitions

The only way to *guarantee* transitions will go smoothly is to never make changes. Since that is unrealistic . . .

• Keep the number of transitions in each child's life to a minimum. If transition must occur, keep previous routines, environments, and adults predictable and in place for as long as possible.

• Trust children and adults to manage transitions constructively and in a timely manner. Transitions are a part of life and can teach worthwhile lessons, especially when they are infrequent and well-planned.

Before a transition

• Through individual conferences, open houses, bulletin board memos, newsletters, email, and flyers, prepare all adults for the coming transition.

• Involve families in planning and keep them informed. Offer them choices and make them a part of decision-making conversations.

• Devise a way that the adults can react to anticipated challenges and generate possible solutions in writing.

• Prepare children for coming changes. Don't talk too much about the future, but do plan

several weeks of preparation and informal visiting to help them ease into their new classroom or group.

• Caution everyone to expect such typical child reactions as challenging behaviors, withdrawal, anger, sadness. Caregivers and parents too may feel these emotions. Emphasize that all these reactions are normal in periods of change and grief.

• Allow for sadness, but don't dwell on it. Help everyone focus on the adventure ahead as soon as they seem ready and willing.

• Keep visits to a future classroom short, simple, and predictable, especially at first. Keep visits upbeat and positive. Lengthen visits slowly, letting children demonstrate their readiness for longer duration.

• Talk with older children about how they might miss a familiar person or place even though they are enjoying a new situation.

• Avoid overlapping transitioning groups, at least at the beginning of the transition period. For example, let younger children who are moving to a new room visit the space with their new teacher at a time when the older children who are still occupying the room are absent.

Relationships, the Heart of Quality Care

Her surprised mother asked her why, and she responded, "I don't want to go to their school. I want to stay with [her caregivers] Lynn and Mike."

No one had thought to prepare her for the fact that [all the children her age were] going to be leaving our familiar nest in a few weeks. The adults assumed she understood—she had been [making yearly transitions] at our center since she was a baby, after all! Luckily her mother was able to set up a visit to the new school *and* another test. That time Serena passed, of course, with flying colors, after she was helped—by all of us—to understand and manage this important transition.

Most young children are not as articulate as Serena was about their reluctance to change. Constructive transitions can take many forms, but the need for thoughtful planning can never be overrated or

• Make it easy for parents to feel part of the transition—participating on a daily basis, if possible. For example, have parents drop off each morning and/or pick up each afternoon in the future classroom.

• Offer children and adults creative opportunities to express their grief as well as celebrate changes ahead. Create class books, tapes, murals, songs, or dramatic enactments about moving, changing, growing up, and fears and expectations. Adult openness makes it safe for children to explore their feelings openly as well.

• Plan a final group gathering of children and adults to facilitate closure.

During a transition

• Make changes slowly, in small steps—especially when the child enters care.

• Set transitions at predictable, regular times, with clear implementation plans. Consider individual needs and temperaments in each plan.

• As much as possible, move groups of children and their primary caregivers to new classrooms as a unit.

• Make children a part of their moving process. Have them choose and carry favorite toys or games to the new classroom. Use familiar pictures and name labels to welcome them into the new space.

After a transition

• Pay attention to things children continue to do in the old way. These instances may signal that change has occurred too fast.

• Create opportunities for children to visit beloved caregivers they have left, until they no longer need to do so. Set up natural ways to maintain loving contact—such as on the playground or during visits to former classrooms. Think in terms of adjustment rather than loss.

• Expect a degree of messiness and confusion for quite a while—sometimes two steps forward, one step back. Avoid the temptation to push children—or adults—faster than they can go; don't encourage anyone to deny his or her true feelings to make it seem easier.

• Be particularly patient, compassionate, and kind. It may take as much as six to eight weeks before everyone is completely settled in and ready to fully participate in the new setting.

dismissed. It is key to helping children, families, and staff let go and move forward—whether it is their first or fifth transition in child care.

Transitions that don't go well are often the result of adults not understanding fundamental principles of child attachment and development. A center director explains,

> I tell my staff that bonding and attachments are what children need—and all of us, for that matter—for resilience and ongoing mental health. Yes, attachment has usually been reserved for family members and kin-like friends, and bonding to temporary caregivers is uncharted territory. Yes, [securely attached] children have a harder time disengaging, and they fuss when their special caregivers are not around. Yes, attachment can be messy, and some people might take advantage of the [close] relationships formed when changes are infrequent. But young children cannot turn their need for attachment off and on, and we shouldn't ask them to try. We have to encourage children to bond to just a few primary caregivers—along with their parents, of course—even if it makes it harder to disengage when the time comes.

Some caregivers and parents might argue that children who experience frequent transitions have fewer problems—citing as evidence that such children have milder reactions and protest less than some others do. The adults might say something like, "It's good for children to learn to be resilient, because life is full of changes. They're going to have to learn to get used to it." But weak reactions to transitions can indicate that children were never strongly attached to their caregivers in the first place, bringing along a host of other developmental problems.

Developmental research (including that described in **A Look at Adult-Child Attachment,** in **Chapter 1,** as well as Lally 1998; Lally, Mangione, & Signer 2002; Ornish 1998; Packard Foundation 2000; Parlakian & Seibel 2002; Perry 1999; Zero to Three 1992) tells us a lot about problems of detachment: Detached children focus on survival, order, and predictability—functions of the lower regions of the brain— as they try to meet their own needs in a world of undependable adults. Regular disruption of important bonds causes children to become manipulative and aggressive and inhibits development of their sense of love and belonging. Their brain development is affected, as is their ability to learn and think. Detachment also makes impulse control more difficult, and that has direct implications for the development of conscience. So even if things might seem fine on the surface, research and experience tells us that they're not.

Regular disruptions in relationships keep children from experiencing the kinds of bonds that become templates for warm, responsive, stable friendships, marriages, and job collegiality as adults. Parents of

Regular disruption of important bonds causes children to become manipulative and aggressive and inhibits development of their sense of love and belonging.

Relationships, the Heart of Quality Care

older children and veteran caregivers know that love, secure attachment, bondedness, is what makes people *more* able to form new relationships and handle other changes—not less. As St. Augustine wrote, "It is better to have loved and lost than to have never loved at all." Staff and families who understand children's developmental needs know that children must be loved in order to thrive as they grow.

Some center staff work as a team to develop thoughtful plans for transition and continuity. Another convinced director reports,

> We have implemented continuity of care, and we've had to do a lot of self-education. We have monthly discussions on brain development, attachments, disengaging from attachments, and coping with grief—the children's and our own. We have a long way to go, but we're working together to understand the danger of detachment. We're trying to clarify our own goals.

For centers working on transitions, **Strategies for Orchestrating Smooth Transitions** (on pages 126–127) offers more ideas.

Day-to-day conversations between a child's regular caregivers and parents are part of what makes that child's care seamless.

Strategy #5: Schedules that put relationship priorities first

Staff scheduling is a complicated challenge under any circumstances. Most child care programs are open from 6 A.M. until 6 P.M., Monday through Friday—that's 12 hours a day, 60 hours a week. Full-time staff typically work only 8-hour days and 40-hour weeks. That resulting gap poses several challenges. Among them: How to set work hours so that the teachers who are responsible for children during the day also are available to parents. And how to support children whose hours in care exceed their caregiver's work shift.

Some centers use floaters or staff from other rooms to cover the time when the children's regular caregivers are gone. Some "telescope" children, juggling them from room to room as daily attendance waxes and wanes. Both solutions seem necessary and efficient to a director looking at the challenge through a logistics lens. But through a relationship-based lens, they are disruptive and ignore the detrimental effects of a daily caregiver-go-round.

In relationship-based care, children are not juggled; staff and schedules are managed so that the needs of children remain the primary focus for everyone. Young children need consistency. Families need regular, ongoing opportunities to get to know, exchange information with, and bond with the person who is their child's regular caregiver. For most parents that means at drop-off and pick-up times.

Benefits of schedules that put relationship priorities first

For children. Day-to-day conversations between a child's regular caregivers and parents are part of what makes that child's care seamless. When a child hears his favorite adults talk about him with pride and he can sense the cooperative spirit between them, he feels loved and safe. When a caregiver's workday starts early or ends late, the child who arrives early or stays late gets calm, one-on-one time with her that he doesn't have to share with other children on more typical schedules. An older child might be invited to help the teacher open or close the classroom; an infant can enjoy being fed with undivided eye contact. Such opportunities for one-on-one interactions can enrich relationships. Children may not be able to speak about how they feel when they are herded or juggled or telescoped for the convenience of staff, but they experience the difference. Most let it be known through their behavior.

For families. When a primary caregiver is present at drop-off or pick-up time, parents can get an accurate idea of what their child did during the day. They can hear anecdotes about toddler Elijah's interactions with friends, the things baby Jason played with, or the discovery 5-year-old Sara made on the playground. A teacher's verbal account gives a more complete picture than do written notes about meals or diaper changes. With meaningful daily interactions with caregivers, families feel good about their choice of care; they know for certain that their children spend time with adults who know them and pay attention to them.

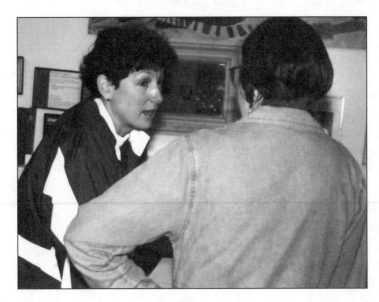

For caregivers. Caregivers benefit from thoughtful scheduling too. Nontraditional hours or a four-day work week offers time a caregiver can plan on for her own family, further education, or personal pursuits. Scheduling a regular caregiver at either end of the day keeps classroom routines stable and materials in order. Daily contact with the adults who share children's care makes a caregiver's job easier, more rewarding, and more fun. Teachers learn things about the children, about their families, and about themselves. The short, informal conversations enrich everyone's lives and offer insights into day-to-day behavior. Deeper relationships with parents and children encourage caregiver retention. When their workday starts early or ends late and only a few children are around, caregivers can be more relaxed as they gear up or wind down for the day. As it is for a parent with several children, being alone with just one child can be a treasured delight—for the adult, as well as the child. Often it is such moments that we keep in our hearts, a hidden benefit of caregiving that can last a lifetime.

For directors and centers. When parents and primary caregivers talk together on a regular basis, crises that require a director's involvement are less likely. Parents can get an immediate explanation for that scratch or bite mark from the equally concerned teacher who was there to see it happen. Small problems are unknotted on a daily basis, keeping directors free to focus on more critical challenges. Also, as always, when caregivers and parents are happy, turnover is lower.

Moving toward schedules that put relationship priorities first

Ideally, center schedules allow a child's caregiver to greet parents every day at drop-off and pick-up times. But like any business, child care centers are subject to labor laws that stipulate time-and-a-half for hours worked over 40. Budget constraints usually make it impossible to cover all hours of operation with a single shift of teachers, even if they were willing to work overtime. One accredited urban center meets the scheduling challenge by staggering staff work hours. Says its director,

> I used to hire floaters to cover the hours at the end of the day, but the turnover rate was very high for these part-time workers and it wasn't good for children and families. I knew I had to do something, but I wasn't sure what. My regular staff didn't want to work 12 hours a day, and [I couldn't afford for them to work] a 60-hour week if they wanted to.
>
> We began to see a way to resolve the problem when one of the regular caregivers offered to come in at 6 A.M., when the first child arrives, in order to leave at 3 P.M. It was good for her because she had a school-age child and wanted to be home in the afternoon. Her coworker was willing to come in at 9 A.M. and work until 6 P.M. That got us started, and that's the way we do it now in all of our classrooms.

This director still hires floaters to support her regular caregiving teams when enrollments go up and the center must meet required

"I used to hire floaters to cover the hours at the end of the day, but the turnover rate was very high for these part-time workers and it wasn't good for children and families."

staff-child ratios; but the floaters don't replace caregivers. This solution makes at least one of the children's two regular caregivers always available to children and to parents. The director adds,

> Problems come up of course, but overall the staff likes it. They like to share stories about the child's day with someone who really wants to know what happened. Parents like it too, for the same reason. Sometimes parents are too busy to stay and chat, but a few words make a difference.

Another program's director encourages her staff to work 10-hour shifts four days a week to cover the hours and support one another as primary caregivers. She explains,

> Some teachers work Monday through Thursday, and some work Tuesday through Friday. . . . They work hard, but they like having a four-day week. It gives them more time with their own families or to do errands. The three-day weekend attracts a lot of people to work in our program.
>
> Both [caregivers on a team] are there at drop-off and pick-up times three days a week, and one is there on each of the other two days. It isn't perfect, but it's better than what we did before. I couldn't keep floaters for early morning or late afternoon shifts. They'd get other jobs, and I'd have to start all over again. Now my part-timers work full days twice a week. Many also substitute for us. It's win-win all around!

Several centers that we observed hire full-time floaters and use them in creative ways to increase quality and continuity. One large program hires well-trained, experienced caregivers as floaters and assigns them to clusters of classrooms, usually one to preschoolers,

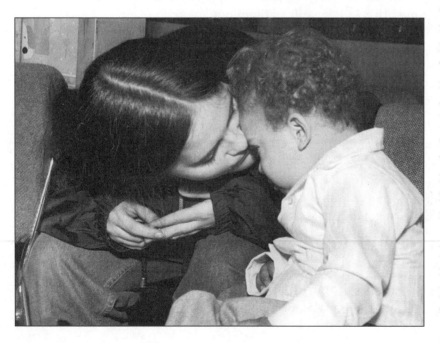

one to toddlers, and one to infants. The floaters move from room to room within their cluster, relieving regular caregivers for lunch breaks or meetings each day. When a caregiver in the cluster is out and needs a substitute, the floaters are the director's first choice.

These floaters are hired with an eye toward fulfilling the additional purpose of offering enrichment experiences

Relationships, the Heart of Quality Care

to the children and mentoring the teachers in their cluster. Although it is expensive to keep extra experienced staff on the payroll, this director is never in a pickle when a regular caregiver calls in sick. The children don't have to deal with a parade of unfamiliar substitutes and part-timers. This helps relationships to blossom over time. The floaters develop authentic bonds with children and parents in their cluster—which keeps them committed to the job. And when a regular caregiver position opens, the director can hire someone whom everyone already knows, increasing continuity for everyone.

No single solution will work for every center. But centers committed to stable, predictable caregiving find their own ways to move ahead and put children's needs first. Of course, there will always be someone eager to explain why adjusting schedules or staffing arrangements is a bad idea.

"Don't bother, they all leave eventually." Even the most creative, carefully planned staffing and coverage scheme is vulnerable to disruption. Caregivers leave for higher paying jobs, they get sick, they want to go back to school or have a baby of their own. But as we have shown, bondedness minimizes the incentive to bolt. When changes do occur, they are often in conjunction with natural transitions rather than in reaction to workplace frustrations.

"We can't have caregivers talking to parents." It may be true that some caregivers are inexperienced or seem too young to understand the nuances of adult relationships. They can say too much, breach confidentiality, get caught up in gossip, or be intimidated by manipulative parents. Occasionally a caregiver might get immersed in adult conversation and forget to supervise the children. And now and then a caregiver becomes possessive of children, and this attitude shows through to parents. All these things, and more, can cause wary directors to keep caregiver-parent conversations to a minimum and control with them in the office.

Savvy veteran directors, however, prepare their staff members and see caregiver-parent conversations as growth opportunities. One director, who admits she doesn't have time to monitor every conversation, says,

> I hire strong communicators who have a grasp of best practice, and assign each one to just a few families. I bring in workshops that increase everyone's skills in relating to parents—and to each other. The workshops always cover things like gossip and confidentiality and conflict resolution. I usually learn a lot too. I see my staff as professional colleagues,

Additional Strategies for Programs Making Children Their Priority

Begin by discussing together the needs of young children in general. Allow yourselves to dream. Imagine there were no regulatory, budget, or staff constraints. Think about what is found naturally in a caring home: small, mixed-age groups of children reared by experienced, loving adults who remain with the children over many years. With that model in mind . . .

Follow a few children around for a day or so, taking notes.

• How many transitions must they go through every day?

• How many different adults must they cope with?

• Are they ever rebuffed or ignored, left to fend for themselves?

• Does each child have one caregiver who is likely to notice if that child is withdrawn, hurt, or being harassed by other children?

Using your observational data, explore the following:

• Are children's needs being met quickly and with compassion?

• Where are there holes or snags in best practice and good care?

• Which behavior management issues might be the result of group size or bumpy transitions?

• Which practices might be keeping attachment bonds from forming or deepening?

• If you were one of those children, what would you say is working? What would you change to have your needs met more effectively?

Examine current program practices.

• Explore what can be done immediately to meet children's needs more effectively. Discuss which areas will require procedures, policies, or more funds.

• Think about what policies and procedures would allow your center to achieve that loving family model. Consider child-centered practices such as small groups, primary caregiving, and continuity of care.

• Look at ways to make scheduling and staffing assignments reflect children's needs rather than adult convenience.

• Pay attention to hidden impacts of adult-centered or finances-driven practices, such as juggling children from room to room as daily attendance waxes and wanes ("telescoping").

• Develop policies that eliminate herding of children and times when children have lengthy waits.

Help parents and staff understand children's need to form secure attachments with caring adults.

• Look at the program's current practices through a relationship lens.

• Celebrate practices that meet attachment needs.

Differentiate children's needs from those of family and center staff.

• Look at situations from different angles. For example, a challenging child sometimes benefits from time away from an anxious parent; on the other hand, the behavior may mean the child and the parent aren't getting *enough* time together.

• Encourage openness about separation anxiety. Consider the possibility that if a parent is deeply distressed and has a choice, it may best for the child to be cared for at home for a while.

• Help parents match their children (and themselves) with settings that allow them to thrive. Consider each child's age, personality, and temperament. Some children do better in centers; some do better in family child care homes; others do best one-on-one with a nanny or a family member.

and I try to give my new people a chance to make mistakes without a lot of backlash—that's how we all learn, isn't it? I keep myself approachable, available to unravel the messes, and I try to notice when someone has said something particularly constructive. . . . What else can you do?

There are no easy answers to the scheduling-staffing-coverage challenge. But from our observations, centers that make thoughtful decisions about scheduling share certain characteristics. The most successful follow three simple rules to meet the needs of children:

- Keep each child's daily schedule simple.
- Limit the number of people involved with each child each day.
- Make continuity a factor when making decisions about part-time staff and substitutes.

In addition, it is important that directors and other staff members are well-versed in developmentally appropriate approaches, brain development, and best practice. They also should have a common vision of what it takes for children to thrive over time. This knowledge promotes well-informed, thoughtful decision making about scheduling.

Every journey begins with a single step

We know it is not possible to reverse decades of entrenched early childhood practice with a few suggestions and stories of successful programs of primary caregiving and continuity of care. Each director and staff member must figure out how to prioritize the needs of children before the work of change can begin in earnest. Each of us has to look at our own priorities and ask, situation by situation, whether we are doing the best we can for the children. Are we making *them* the priority?

Putting children's needs first is not always easy. Not even for this early childhood educator with more than 10 years of experience as a center director—a woman who had always thought that children were her number-one priority:

> One day in walks a young mother with her 2-year-old son . . . . I took her on a tour of the building and we talked about napping, food, fees, hours— all the usual things. She said she was concerned about her child's transition to child care, and I explained that children sometimes cry when their parents leave, but most of them get used to the center in a few days. Our staff is trained to help. As she was leaving, she asked if she could watch the toddlers for a few minutes.

The director told her she could, and returned to her office without thinking anymore about it. But two hours later a child psychologist who worked as a consultant for the center came to see her in her office.

> The psychologist said she had found the mother and child crying in the hallway. The young woman was distraught at the thought of separating from her son. Her parents 1were telling her that it was time for her to go back to work; her husband was leaving the decision up to her. But she didn't think she was ready.
>
> I felt confused. I said to the psychologist, "We run a good center. He'll be fine." But that didn't satisfy her. "If the mother is unhappy it will be very hard for the child," she argued. Finally I asked her, what does *she* think I should do? She looked me in the eye and said, "You should encourage the mom to stay home." I told her I'd think about it.

The director had no intention of making a phone call to the mother. Her center's enrollment was low and she wanted to fill the slot. If she didn't get more children, she was going to have to lay off staff. All afternoon she kept busy, distracting herself from thinking about the problem. She knew the psychologist was right; it was better for the *child* if the mother stayed home until she was ready.

> I never thought the day would come when I would discourage a parent from coming to my center, but that's what happened. The next morning I called the mother; I even talked to the grandparents and convinced them to support the mother's decision. . . . I still think about that family. I can't cover the cost of running a center if I don't have the children. But the question is, Why am I in the child care business if I'm not helping children?

As this director discovered, putting children's needs first is not always an easy decision. But it is one that some directors and center staff do make, as the stories in this chapter make clear. **Additional Strategies for Programs Making Children Their Priority** (see page 134) suggests ways for centers to keep the focus on the children—especially infants, toddlers, and children with special needs.

◆ ◆ ◆

In this chapter we described five important strategies for developing workplace and child care practices, with an aim toward delivering high-quality care to children in the center setting. In **Chapter 5,** the third and last of our "solutions" chapters, we offer strategies to foster a sense of community among the adults who share children's care.

5

Building a Caring Community
around Children

One of the primary goals of relationship-based care is to surround children with a *community* of caring adults (parents, caregivers/teachers, and directors) who interact as partners or friends. Relationships go beyond typical norms for customers and service providers, employers and employees, supervisors and subordinates. The warm bonds that form between adults make them more comfortable sharing the care and putting the needs of the children first. They are willing to support policies such as primary caregiving and low ratios, even if these approaches cost a little more. They value each connection in the parent-caregiver-child and director-parent-caregiver triads. Working together on each child's behalf, these family-like communities encourage secure attachments and seamless care.

Relationship-based programs employ many different strategies to build community. They embrace the family model for adult relationships as well as for interactions between adults and children. They share power and work through the challenges of close relationships, rather than ignore them. They send caregivers regularly to visit children's homes. They welcome families into the classroom. They plan activities that give parents and caregivers opportunities to relax together and get better acquainted. When interpersonal issues threaten the quality of care, these programs bring in specialists and consultants for advice.

Once relationships between adults are understood and valued as an important element of quality in child care settings, the possibilities (both formal and informal) for creating community are endless. The following strategies offer some places to start.

Strategy #1: The family model

Our field of early care and education is just beginning to understand the family model of child care and its emphasis on close, caring relationships. In too many centers the business and elementary-school models still dominate, with their focus on hierarchy, productivity, efficiency, and inclination to define people by their "jobs" rather than by how they relate to others. In the business model, the director's job is to make sure the center meets licensing regulations and is fully enrolled. She supervises staff and puts out each day's inevitable fires. Teachers receive direction from the director and are expected to follow regulations, attend training, and perform duties assigned to them in the classroom. Parents are the consumers; their role is to pay for services provided. Children and their needs take a back seat to financial and staffing considerations. Relationships are secondary, cordial but formal.

This model may be good for business, but it is inappropriate for raising young children. Research and experience show that if we want young children to thrive, they must be in places where the adults *care* about them and about one another. Childrearing is a time-consuming, messy process. For best results, human needs for bonding and attachment must be everyone's primary concern.

The goal of relationship-based centers is to operate like a well-functioning, extended family. Under the family model, children are not the "product" of a child care program, families are more than consumers of services, and staff members are more than service providers. Instead, adults are encouraged to participate in a human community, which forms gradually as caring, comfort, and trust develop over time. In relationship-based centers, directors, caregivers, support staff, and families recognize and value one another's gifts, their interdependency, and the love they share for the children. They dedicate themselves to creating strategies that build cooperative circles of love and care that benefit everyone.

Benefits of the family model

For children. In the family model of care, long-term connections rather than short-lived ones are the norm. Important relationships that are sustained over a period of years enable children to develop and function at their highest level and give them a lasting image of what it is like to be part of a community that cares. Children in relationship-based centers develop the expectation that they will be valued and attached to others, a template they will use throughout their lives.

For families. Programs following the family model offer parents and other family members a home away from home. The community circle is wide and multi-generational, welcoming siblings and grandparents. Family-like connections offer a safe haven from stress-filled, results-driven work lives. Relationship-based centers are comfortable places where parents can go to enjoy the company of their own children, the children of friends, and other adults with whom they can share childrearing's joys and challenges.

Inside this caring community, adults feel comfortable entering into a healthy give-and-take about childrearing values. They can observe and learn new skills from one another, as parents in earlier generations learned from extended families and friends before interpersonal connections became so fragmented. Parents who feel supported and cared about by staff and other parents are able to shift out of work mode; they feel empowered to partner with caregivers and to think rationally about shared goals. The caring connections forged with staff members and other families may continue over many years. These relationships and their authentic bonds of community contribute to everyone's mental health.

For caregivers. High-quality caregivers thrive in the family model. A caregiver's natural tendency to bond is valued and supported by families and directors alike. They aren't told to "leave the parents alone"; instead they can act on their instincts and make a phone call or visit when needed. Challenges that arise over childrearing are easier to overcome. They don't need to hide or discount the bonds that develop naturally with the children and with other adults. Strong, healthy connections are encouraged between caregivers and parents, as well as among coworkers; community is the norm. Comfortable relationships between adults become incentives for caregivers to stay on the job. Warmth and responsiveness are part of the daily benefits package for all who work within a high-functioning family model.

For centers and directors. The family model supports directors and centers as much as it does children, families, and staff. Word spreads about centers that have thriving communities. They become known as high quality and family friendly—as good places to work and to bring children for care. They tend to keep staff and families, fill up every year, and maintain waiting lists. A director can be confident in the level of quality her center offers because she knows that all the

Word spreads about centers that have thriving communities. They become known as high quality and family friendly.

adults there are working toward common goals, with children's needs first.

A director's job is never conflict free, but her work of relationship building resembles that within extended families where goodwill and a common vision prevail. As among parents and teachers, deep relationships developed between a director and parents and staff help her feel supported and strong, both personally and professionally.

Moving toward the family model

To create community, centers must keep their focus on child-centered, relationship-based care. Successful centers encourage a network of reciprocal connection similar to that found in the family model of adult relationships. There are many "right" ways to help relationships thrive while keeping a comfortable sense of boundaries. Each center will arrive at its own formula for success. Relationship-based programs generally set aside time for staff to sort out the details and evaluate policies as they go along. Such forums to discuss and establish a shared approach give staff an opportunity to strengthen their own relationships. Conversations get challenges out in the open and allow the adults to respond to challenging circumstances. Explains one director,

> Family members inherit the structure, but we have to create it. For example, we have found it better to encourage parents to move along in the mornings and hang out in the afternoons. It is actually mentioned in our policies as part of our expectations. We allow a few weeks of transition, but after that we nudge parents out the door to keep our morning routines flowing smoothly. Because we have it in the policies, we rarely have to do much to enforce it. Parents understand and see it as a help to all of us. We put out extra snacks at pick-up time, and that is when we work on casual conversations and building relationships.

Another center might do this differently. The important thing is to think through the strategies together. A center-wide policy might make sense in some situations; age-based policies might work for others. What counts is a thoughtful, planned, even-handed approach communicated clearly, in advance, so that everyone feels counted in the mix. It helps to have written policies that can be shared when teachers begin a new relationship with parents. Experienced caregivers can mentor novices too.

Relationship-based programs that successfully promote the family model offer us starting points for working through arguments such as these:

"Closeness causes trouble." Knowing that bonding is good for children, early care and education professionals tend to accept as constructive a certain amount of friendliness between the adults caring for young children. But some, including some parents, find the notion of encouraging close adult relationships to be asking for trouble. They believe that anytime close relationships form, especially if they turn into friendships, the potential for hurt feelings and anger will lurk in the form of cliques, favoritism, manipulation. Challenges can surface over all kinds of issues—children's birthday celebrations, gift exchanges, dinner invitations, phone calls after hours. If handled badly, each offers potential for people to feel slighted or misunderstood.

Centers that value relationship-based care don't try to dodge the challenges by rejecting the family model. Instead they reflect on the dynamics of authentic relationships, share experiences, and learn from their successes as well as their mistakes. Relationship-based centers develop sensitive, flexible ways to keep things feeling balanced for every member in the group; they think through policies and systems for dealing with grievances so that they are ready when difficulties arise.

"It's hard to be fair." Evenhandedness is critical to juggling multiple relationships constructively. Policies can recognize that some relationships inevitably will be closer than others. An evenhanded approach encourages the same kind of discretion, concern for other people's feelings, and confidentiality that considerate adults show to one another in their churches, families, and neighborhoods. For example, a policy can remind caregivers to give equal attention to all families at drop-off and pick-up times, to avoid showing favoritism by talking too much with one family over the rest. The bottom line inside the center is to offer the same options and attention to every family, regardless of personal feelings of closeness.

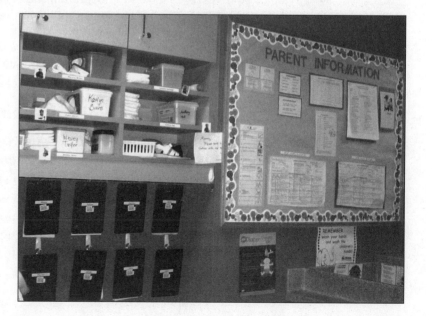

Fairness can be demonstrated in many different ways. Take birthday parties, for example: An *inappropriate* approach would be for a caregiver to refuse invitations from all children except those of her special friends and to talk about it in front of other families. Deciding in advance how to approach the challenge of birthdays helps to avoid this kind of insensitivity. One teacher might encourage families to hold their children's birthday parties at the center; another teacher might prefer to celebrate each child's birthday at the center in a similar way, with the parents as honored guests but not sponsors; a third teacher might set up home visits around the time of each child's birthday and might or might not also attend home parties. In relationship-based centers, thoughtful, sensitive teachers help those less sophisticated find an appropriate, professional balance in their daily interactions with families, so that everyone feels part of the circle.

"Parents will walk all over us." The same caring impulse that makes caregivers so good at connecting with children and families also leaves them vulnerable to pressure—innocent or manipulative—for special favors. When "*stop being a doormat!*" is too hard to follow, the business model's strict policies against fraternizing with families can seem very appealing. Centers using the family model have policies that are clear and firm but also *flexible*—more like an air pillow than a rock. Explains one director,

> We don't want to [rewrite the rules] for every parent, but we also stay open to possibilities. We are like a good family and keep "win-win" as our goal. We try to look for cooperation and collaboration rather than lock-step "obedience." . . . I went to an inspirational self-esteem workshop a long time ago. What the presenter said has stayed with me, "Firmness shows that you respect yourself; kindness shows that you respect the other." You be both firm and kind at the same time.

Strategy #2: A sense of community

Some may think creating community in a workplace is too difficult, but in most child care centers it can happen quite naturally, especially when directors set the tone. Relationship skills are taught as much by example as by instruction. Directors who value community know that the *way* they perform daily tasks is as important as what they accomplish. A dedication to openness, a willingness to listen, empathy, compassion, honesty, and strong professional ethics are at the heart of that work.

Relationships, the Heart of Quality Care

It is usually the director who clarifies each person's role in the center's community and inspires collaboration. A relationship-based director values each adult's position in the group and tries to understand both the caregiver and parent points of view. Her respect and warm concern—for the adults on her staff as well as for those who use the center's services—becomes a model for all to follow.

A director who communicates her ideas and values in an honest and easy way, and who encourages other adults to do the same, strengthens the director-caregiver-parent triad. Such a director permits people to talk about their troubles, their hopes, and their dreams. She allows everyone to explore solutions to challenges, and rallies the group when times are hard. Teachers, support staff, and parents reciprocate by valuing the director's work and by cooperating as a team. They support the director with suggestions as well as compliments, and lighten her load by taking on responsibilities and looking for solutions to problems on their own. Mutual support like this empowers adults to build trusting relationships and create community. Day by day they create a circle of respect and care for one another. The center takes on a family-like feel, and everyone—adult and child alike—looks forward to returning again and again.

Of course, no community is perfect or conflict free. But challenges *can* be seen as cause for celebration. The closer our relationships are with others, the more comfortable we are being ourselves; the more deeply we care, the greater the possibility that strong feelings will come out. However, when we are dedicated to cooperation and community building, interpersonal problems become more manageable. Sometimes directors have to help navigate issues; other times staff and parents can untangle issues alone. A sense of community gives its members the courage they need to be honest and the strength to work things through.

A sense of community gives everyone the courage they need to be honest and the strength to work things through.

Benefits of a sense of community

For children. Children benefit from a warm, positive adult community because their world feels seamless; what is practiced by the adults in one setting is practiced—or at least understood—by the adults in the other. They don't feel confused or get tangled up in loyalty conflicts as they try to meet divergent expectations. Children also benefit by watching their significant adults interact. Following the adults' example, children can learn to listen, feel empathy, exhibit patience, act assertively, and treat others with kindness and respect.

For families. When center staff demonstrate positive relationship skills, they set the tone for every interaction. Parents learn that relaxed, friendly, and reasonable interaction is the norm, regardless of how upset or confused they might feel. Their interactions with the various members of the staff are balanced, no matter how close they feel toward a few. The example of professionalism set by the center's staff encourages parents to communicate assertively when they are distressed or concerned. They can relax in the knowledge that they will be heard. In the family model, each parent's skill in building community is appreciated, fortified, and used to help everyone grow.

For caregivers. Caregivers' jobs are less stressful when the director has good relationship skills and community building is a center-wide goal. A relationship-focused director eases conflicts with parents and supports caregivers who are doing their job well. This toddler teacher describes what happens when those skills are lacking:

> In the center where I used to work, an older brother of one of the children came into the room. He got excited and pushed one of the little children, and that child got hurt. I told the center director and she suggested that I tell the mother to drop off the older child first [before coming to the toddler room]. I did, but the mother was very upset. She acted as though I was expelling her child from the whole day care. She was so upset that she stopped talking to me. When the director heard about this, she made me apologize. . . . The director was the kind of person who avoided conflict, and so she didn't want to talk with the parent herself. The parent continued to send the child and we talked now and then, but she stopped making eye contact.

It takes skill to know how to support parents as well as caregivers when conflicts arise. Relationship-based directors have learned to listen to parents and take their concerns seriously without devaluing the caregiver's experience. Caregivers benefit because they know the director will support them, even when they run into obstacles. They can trust the director will take time to understand their concerns. A caregiver is not abandoned in favor of an emotional parent.

Caregivers also benefit from a community in which staff are encouraged to talk openly about their own mistakes and learn from them. Self-examination isn't always easy. This thoughtful director came to understand that her own need for close connection was adversely affecting parent-caregiver ties:

> I never thought much about my role as director until I [prepared to take] a leave for a summer to go to graduate school. Before I left, I replaced myself with an assistant director. My goal, I thought, was to enable her

to have as deep a connection with the parents as I had. . . . One day, late in the spring, I stood near the front door looking for Timmy's mom. We always had a good conversation when she was leaving the center. When I didn't see her, I asked my assistant where she was. She told me that Timmy and his mom had already left. I was crushed! Tim's mom had said goodbye to my assistant and not to me! I felt unhappy and left out, even though everything was working out as I'd hoped. I was surprised to realize that I didn't want my assistant to have the important relationships with the families.

I understand now why it can be so hard for directors like me to tell parents that their most important relationship is with their child's teacher! Sometimes, I guess, I undercut the parent-caregiver relationship or make it seem less important than it is.

This director realized that to support strong parent-caregiver ties, she had to rein in her own impulse to be everybody's best friend. The caregivers in her center benefited because in sharing her revelations with the staff, she made it safe for them to be close to parents *and* to explore personal challenges more openly within the collegial circle.

For centers and directors. An experienced director walks a narrow line between supporting parents and supporting caregivers. If she loses her balance, her safety net is her strong relationships with her staff and her ability to communicate. As one teacher recalls,

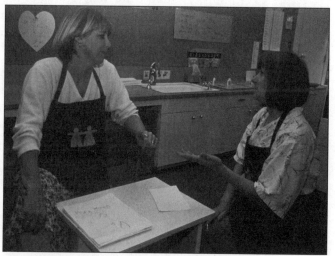

I got a note from my director saying that a new child would be enrolling in my classroom the following morning. All she told me was his name and his date of birth. I was upset, because she didn't tell me anything about the child or the family. So I went to the director and asked what else she knew. She was apologetic; she realized she'd been careless. As it turned out this was to be the child's first experience at a center.

Everything went smoothly, but it worked out that way because I had the information I needed. I was able to get it because the director and I had a good relationship, and I assumed she'd been distracted when she wrote the note. But if our relationship hadn't been good, I don't know what I would have done. I know I would have resented her and felt the note was demeaning. I might even have taken some of those feelings out on the child—I *know* I wouldn't have made the same effort to welcome him and his mom to the center. My relationship with the director made all the difference.

When directors and staff have deep, positive relationships and communicate effectively, the whole center benefits. The director can trust that small oversights won't turn into confrontations; she can assume that the staff will help out if she forgets or becomes overwhelmed. Everything runs more smoothly because the director breathes more easily. She knows that she can count on staff support— even their willingness to go the extra mile—when help is needed.

Skills that support relationships and collegial community aren't built in a day. But when they are in place, with family as the model, everyone thrives.

Moving toward a sense of community

In relationship-based care, the director is one of many in the circle of caring relationships that surrounds each child in care. Staff are empowered by a director who creates an organizational hierarchy that is flat. Such a director lets teachers know that their opinions matter and that their collegial relationship with her matters too. The director sets a tone of respectful interactions between coworkers by modeling that tone herself. Director-staff respect becomes a template for parent-caregiver relationships.

A director acknowledges and empowers her staff when she gives them opportunities to speak and pays attention to what she hears. This sets the stage for honest conversation and builds rapport. Caregivers are more likely to be open with a supervisor who talks freely about her own shortcomings. Says one director,

> One of the ways I encourage my staff to speak up is by admitting that I make mistakes. The staff sees that I'm pretty comfortable with that. We have standards, and we expect ourselves to measure up, but we make mistakes along the way. It just happens.

This kind of openness is key to turning a center into an authentic, supportive, respectful community.

When teachers and support staff in the child care setting feel empowered, they join in the overall effort to keep improving the quality of care by giving their opinions, offering solutions, and making suggestions. A caregiver in an infant room at a suburban center shares what can happen when caregivers—and parents—believe their voices are heard:

> I thought that the children in my room would be better off if we all moved together at the end of the year. My daughter had been cared for by 13 different caregivers by the time she was 3, and I didn't think that was right

Relationships, the Heart of Quality Care

for children. I asked the parents first, and they liked the idea and so we went to the director. The center didn't mind as long as the parents agreed, and so that fall we *all* moved up. The parents thought it was wonderful. The director was happy.

Empowered caregivers support their director by sharing the responsibility for ensuring center excellence. A director who has good instincts, but is dealing at any given moment with multiple problems big and small, will gladly follow the caregivers' lead when they speak on behalf of children. Here, a director who has worked 15 years at an independent center in Southern California talks about the importance of having staff who are committed to the quality of the program:

> I rely on my staff. I couldn't run this center alone. A few years ago, one of our caregivers wanted to set up a toddler program. We only took care of preschool children then. A group of us met and thought about what we would have to do. Did we need to build a new classroom? What would it look like? Eventually the board of directors got involved. The caregiver who wanted the program worked with the board, and eventually we were able to make it happen. We've had the toddler program three years, and parents love it—we all love it! But we could never have done it if we hadn't been able to work as a team.

The center director's role often can feel thankless. She's responsible for enrollment, quality care, staying within budget, ordering supplies, making sure that parents wishes are being met and that staff are satisfied, covering for surprise absences, developing curriculum, keeping boards and owners in the loop. The burden of management is on her shoulders. Even though they may put on a good face, many directors feel stressed out by the job. "I feel that the aloneness of being a director is a major problem," laments one. "It seems an accomplishment just to have survived another year." But when staff members feel empowered, the job is shared. Directors feel more hopeful, problems are less overwhelming, and responsibilities become more manageable.

It can be unsettling for some directors to involve their staff in decision making and other responsibilities, but directors who make that leap are richly rewarded. Adding parents to the circle tightens the director-caregiver-parent triad, building a community of shared power that is well worth the challenge of putting it into place. Here are some steps toward that goal.

Develop empowerment strategies. Transforming a hierarchical pyramid into a circle of shared power is one of the most effective ways to create community among adults. Many directors begin by inviting caregivers and families to share their thoughts and become involved in

"I feel that the aloneness of being a director is a major problem."

the process of making changes and decisions. Some set up a suggestion box and ask everyone to submit their ideas anonymously. Others use naptime or after-hours conversation circles to explore classroom changes or exchange experiences of successful conflict management. Still others invite adults to come together and talk informally about relationships and power, or they hold formal workshops to increase everyone's understanding of the issues. (**Staff Feel Empowered When...** offers some other ideas.)

One innovative director decided to model cooperation and shared power by hiring a codirector.

> I think codirecting sets the tone for relationship building at a center. My codirector and I work hard at sharing power. It is a little like a marriage. Someone has to give up power; someone has to speak up and ask for power that hasn't been shared. I've had to learn that there are times when I'm still holding onto power. I'm not always aware that's happening.

She welcomes input from staff too.

> This arrangement has had an effect on the staff, because they know I mean it when I say I want to share the power with them too. . . . When staff come to me with a problem, I don't solve it. I ask them what they would do. They have good ideas. If they need information, I tell them where to get it.
>
> Sometimes my codirector and I talk about budget choices with the staff. When we had to decide whether to give staff a pay raise or hire a

---

Staff Feel Empowered When . . .

- **Their ideas are invited and acted upon.** A suggestion box, for example, can help with staff who are shy or hesitant to go out on a limb in front of others.

- **Their contributions are acknowledged publicly.** Always credit the source of good ideas.

- **Problems are dealt with openly.** For example, acknowledge burnout; talk about how to deal with difficult parents or children.

- **They have a concrete idea of what they are trying to accomplish.** New staff often benefit from being assigned a more experienced mentor.

- **They have the authority to solve problems independently.** A classroom team or the entire staff can work on a particular problem to-

gether to recommend solutions and policy suggestions.

- **Classroom issues are teachers' domain unless they request help.** Each caregiver works directly with parents and children in her primary caregiver group, as well as with coworkers in her classroom.

- **They are encouraged to share their innovations or successes,** for example, at meetings and workshops.

- **They have opportunities to learn.** Training staff in assertiveness is useful, as is training directors to empower others.

- **They take workshops together,** for example, a workshop on conflict management or on developing communication skills.

floater, we asked them what they wanted to do. They chose the floater. It didn't matter to us [which one]—we did what the staff suggested.

This director also backs her staff. For example, when the center was invited to participate in a program at a local university,

> It was interesting and well organized, but the instructor called the caregivers *paras* (paraprofessionals). Here we don't have "lead" teachers; we work in teams—no one is under anyone else. The staff were so incensed over the way the instructor described their jobs that they wanted to drop out of the program. It was a good program in other ways, so I tried to win them back by making light of it. . . . They came around, but I can honestly say that I would have quit the program if they had continued to be angry or resistant. I would have supported them.

These strong statements of confidence and support reflect the thinking of a director committed to empowerment and relationship-based care. She is willing to do whatever it takes to turn her center into a community of professionals, working together on behalf of the children.

Directors also empower staff by sharing administrative responsibilities with trusted caregivers, or even with parent volunteers. Some directors assign mentor teachers to work in classrooms; others empower veteran staff as team leaders to oversee groups of classrooms and prevent or settle conflicts among staff. As this director discovered, peer leadership can reduce interpersonal squabbles and improve overall staff morale.

> I was always being asked to step in and resolve personal problems. One caregiver felt threatened by a staff member who was pretty domineering. Then there was the caregiving team in the toddler room. Both of the caregivers were good, but they had different temperaments and styles and kept trying to draw me into their conflicts. My team leaders meet with their caregivers every week and talk about whatever is a problem. These women are patient and kind, and they know what to do. I meet with them and the rest of the staff when no one can figure out a solution. But they handle most of the problems on their own.

Sometimes conflicts are a result of differences in style, personality, beliefs, and family goals; sometimes they arise out of external factors such as physical space, state regulations, or national standards for excellence. Directors don't always have the time or the skill to unravel interpersonal problems one by one. By delegating this responsibility among other experienced staff members, relationship-based directors share the burden as well as the power while building a strong community of colleagues.

A director committed to empowerment and relationship-based care is willing to do whatever it takes to turn her center into a community of professionals, working together on behalf of the children.

Hire independent consultants to navigate snags. Some directors turn to an independent consultant's neutral perspective to help them strengthen relationships. The most effective consultants demonstrate respect for both directors and caregivers as professionals. Staff must know that the consultant values their experience and point of view; directors must feel that the consultant is worth the price. A consultant explains,

> If I take the director's point of view too quickly, the caregivers will feel I've betrayed their trust. The same thing happens if I support the caregivers without hearing what the director has to say. We can't get anywhere without a basic belief in one another and basic trust.

Some consultants use an independent assessment tool in their work, such as the Early Childhood Environment Rating Scale–ECERS (Harms, Clifford, & Cryer 1998a), the Infant Toddler Environment Rating Scale–ITERS (Harms, Clifford, & Cryer 1998c; Harms, Cryer, & Clifford 2003), or the NAEYC accreditation tool (1998, 2004). These rating instruments are particularly important if the consultant is trying to resolve a conflict related to space, materials, or interactions with children. According to one consultant,

> [Assessment tools such as] the ECERS and the ITERS are empowering. You have them as baselines. Caregivers and directors know what they have to do and why and what steps they need to take to make a program better. Caregivers who are less verbal have a tool for explaining what they want—more manipulatives, for example, or books that are in better condition. The ECERS gives directors and caregivers a common reference point and the power to identify and defend their strengths. When I'm not there, they don't have to start from scratch every time they need help.

An effective consultant generally begins at a respectful distance, listening rather than making quick, obvious suggestions. Center staff and parents are acknowledged as knowing the children best. Rather than impose solutions, the consultant helps them come to their own understanding of the issues and their own ways of responding. A good consultant helps strengthen the sense of community among staff and families, and relieves directors and staff of some of the stresses inherent in center life.

Strategy #3: Home visiting

Nothing builds community like sharing our lives with others. This makes home visits as important to the parent-caregiver relationship as they are to the relationship between caregiver and child. Home visits offer adults an opportunity to get to know each other away from the center's distractions. A caregiver's visit to a child's home might be as short as an hour and as long as an afternoon, usually combining a formal interview with casual conversation, perhaps even a meal. Some visits have no agenda and allow for family life to unfold naturally. First-time visitors might begin with a checklist or an informal script to help everyone move more quickly through the awkward shyness that is predictable at the beginning of any relationship. Over time, visits usually become more social. Parents may also begin to use repeat visits as occasions to share questions or concerns they are more comfortable bringing up in the privacy of their own home.

Visits typically offer the caregiver a window into the family's life—an opportunity to observe natural parent-child interactions, meet siblings, get to know the family pet. Her informal observations can identify safety or health issues, developmental challenges, and areas of shared interest worthy of future conversations. She will note whether the home has age-appropriate toys and books, and perhaps finally understand why Steven knows the jingle to so many television commercials. Teacher visits to the family home build a sturdy bridge between home and child care, and the benefits follow child, caregiver, and parent back to the center.

For example, observant caregivers can pattern their interactions with a child after those of the parent. Here, a caregiver explains how she develops a relationship built around the parents' expectations, her own expectations, and the child's personality:

> When I go to the family's home, I spend time with the child on the floor and I talk to the parents. I watch to see how they soothe the baby, how they hold her, feed her, diaper her. Do they burp her over their knee or against their shoulder? Do they rock her when they feed her or sit still? Do they comfort him with words or backrubs? Do they have special toys for the child to hold or look at near the changing table?

Information collected during a visit helps ease the transition from home to child care, by yielding insights on how to help children adjust to being away from home. One caregiver noticed that a baby was accustomed to falling asleep in a portable swing at home.

> We wanted the child's sleep arrangement to feel familiar at the center, so the director and I asked child care licensing to waive the requirement that prohibits the use of swings in centers. They granted us this request, acknowledging that the temporary use of a swing would be a comfort to the child until she could be eased into using a bed. And they understood that it would be less stressful for the parents.

Nothing builds community like sharing our lives with others.

Benefits of home visiting

For children. Imagine having one of your best friends drop by at your home, meeting your family and admiring your favorite things. This is the kind of excitement a child can feel when his teacher comes to visit. Many important things are communicated both verbally and nonverbally. From that time on, mentions of Jack the hamster or *Goodnight Moon* in the nightstand drawer mean something to both caregiver and child. Home visits help create a shared context that enables the caregiver to more quickly understand a child, especially when the child's words are limited. Home visits also offer children emotional benefits similar to that of a family reunion—*"Finally, all the members of my beloved family are in one place."* In the best visits, a child enjoys her favorite adults laughing and talking together, modeling the art of relationship building, and encircling her with relaxed, shared, loving care.

For families. Having "the teacher" visit is a stress for some parents; but home visits can be rich and rewarding anyway, once the ice is broken and adults relax. Families can be themselves in their own space, surrounded by the comforts of home. They also have the opportunity to get to know their child's caregiver in less formal ways and develop the kind of mutual trust that benefits everyone. Removed from the hurried confusion of drop-off and pick-up times, parents see how the caregiver interacts with their child and the warm responsiveness that has evolved between them. Families can delight in observing that

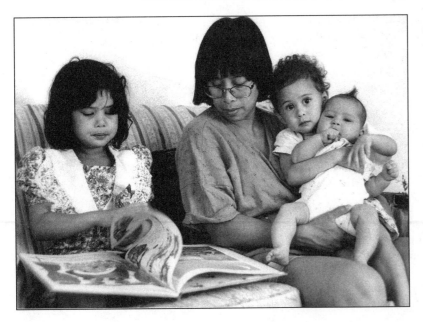

there is someone else who sees how special their child really is.

Also, parents feel acknowledged when a nonjudgmental caregiver shows interest in their personal lives. Once the channel of communication opens, adults find things in common that go beyond children and child care. Questions and worries are easier to bring up. Relaxed conversation becomes a comfortable norm.

For caregivers. Whatever their feelings about home visits beforehand, caregivers typically report glowing successes once a round of visits is complete. Seeing families in their home environments gives a caregiver insights and understandings rarely discovered any other way. She sees with new eyes the shy, reserved father playing a joyful game of hide-and-seek with his toddler. Watching Grandma gently rock the baby and sing a heart-filled lullaby, she now understands why Haider fusses at the center when he is put down for a nap. Big brothers poking and teasing Raul helps her to understand his wariness during free play. Observing Jayla's quiet life with PaPa and Mr. Cat explains the child's fear of noise and strangers.

In addition to invaluable observations, home visits offer calm, focused opportunities for teachers to reach out and respond to parents. Once everyone gets beyond any discomfort they might feel about a visit with someone they hardly know, the concern they share for the child opens the way for a caring adult relationship to flourish. And, of course, relationships are what make quality care flourish too.

For centers and directors. In centers where home visits are a regular part of the program, it is our observation that relationships among adults seem noticeably stronger. Parents and caregivers seek each other out for daily chats and laugh with an easy camaraderie. Complaints are reduced and problems are resolved with less fanfare, often without involvement by the director. Directors reap the benefits in decreased turnover and increased empowerment and professionalism. People are *at home* with one another at the center, and quality care is enhanced simply by the comfort they feel in one another's presence.

Moving toward home visiting

Some programs make home visiting a requirement. In Head Start, caregivers or family support workers are expected to make at least two home visits per year; in Early Head Start (for children birth to 3) visits might occur more often. In some of these programs, when a child enrolls, a family support worker visits the family to develop an individualized "family partnership agreement" that identifies family goals, responsibilities, and she timetables and charts the family's progress. Caseworkers, advocates, or health staff members might accompany caregivers to the home, or caregivers might visit families independently (Head Start Bureau 1999). This family support worker in a bilingual, bicultural Early Head Start program describes her home-visiting experience:

> Home visits offer calm, focused opportunities for teachers to reach out and respond to parents.

I take the partnership agreement with me and [the parents and I] talk about their goals. . . . We talk about steps that they will have to take to be successful. Sometimes they need more information, or they might need someone to drive them to a meeting. One needed help with a child who had Down syndrome; another had a child who had seizures. . . . I check in on parents every two weeks or so, to see how they're doing. When I visit them at their homes they offer me coffee and we sit and talk a while. We get to know each other pretty well. When they don't know what to do or where to go for help, they call me.

In this program, visiting caregivers focus on the child, while the family support worker focuses on the parents. Caregivers and family support staff talk informally and at regularly scheduled meetings about any concerns; the caseworker might even attend parent-caregiver conferences.

Unfortunately, a commitment to home visiting is not universal, even among Head Start programs. Some programs or directors miss its value; some caregivers are too shy or think they are too busy to visit family homes; and a few parents simply say no, because they are too busy or are embarrassed by their homes or are intimidated by someone "in authority" visiting.

There are also insensitive directors who sabotage home visiting by expecting caregivers to make visits after work hours, with no compensation. Such a burden can lead to resentment and resistance. Other directors veto home visits—along with long daily chats and telephone calls between caregivers and parents—because they don't want to "bother" the families or deal with the "complications" that relationships bring. Or they may not have confidence in caregivers' ability to do a good job. Even if home visits are welcomed by parents, supported by directors, and a mandatory part of their work, not every caregiver or caseworker is comfortable going into a family home. Fear of frustration or disappointment can become self-fulfilling prophecy for caregivers whose loud rejection of the idea makes clear they never wanted to visit a home in the first place.

Here are some ideas that programs have come up with to make success more likely.

Go together. In some Head Start programs, caregivers and family support workers make home visits together. They give each other mutual support and can compare notes; plus, going together lets the caregiver-parent relationship develop alongside the one between parent and caseworker. In some programs, a classroom team of caregivers visits together. Traveling with a trusted colleague makes it feel more comfortable to enter an unfamiliar neighborhood or a family's home when the adults are all still strangers. The team approach can be a key to having visits happen at all.

Suggest meeting parents in a neutral place. One Early Head Start program deals with the problem of parents unwilling to open their homes by arranging to meet them at restaurants, libraries, parks, even at a caregiver's own home. The program knows that the spirit of the visiting mandate is to see parents and children informally, outside of the "school" environment. Over the years, this respect-filled attitude has won more than a few parents over to opening the door to home visiting.

Go with a plan. Making successful home visits can seem like a breeze to friendly, experienced caregivers; but there are always some who need help getting started or organized to make it work. Working with fellow teachers to create a visiting plan and/or pairing new home visitors with veteran mentors can ease tensions all around. Plans also help families to understand the value and basic agenda of the visit. Most centers devise a simple letter to send home and post a copy along with sign-up sheets on each classroom door. This gives parents the time they need to digest information and feel at ease if they see home visiting as a new idea.

Some plans include a simple agenda or script to help smooth out the rough spots. A program might suggest home visitors use a short questionnaire or "scavenger hunt" to break the ice. With openers such as "Show me your favorite book" or "What do you do to get ready for bed?" children happily lead the way to easy interactions. In one Georgia center, caregivers take a current developmental checklist to share with parents—not as a "report card" but as a tool to compare observations. It has been their ongoing experience that a parent and a caregiver sometimes observe different things, if only because children show their parents and teachers different sides of themselves. During the home visit, the adults use the checklist together to see what the child does when everyone is in the room.

Budget the cost. At an average of two hours for each visit, the cost of adding home visiting to a program is relatively small. But budgeting for home visits can be a problem for a financially strapped center (especially if the director or teachers also are resistant to the idea). As with many quality initiatives, when a center's staff are committed, a director will find ways to cover costs. Some programs use strategies like those described in **Chapter 4** for overcoming fiscal barriers to continuity of care. They might charge families a set fee at the beginning

> Pairing new home visitors with veteran mentors can ease tensions all around.

of the year to cover staff overtime, or they might use fees from programs less expensive to run, such as school-age child care or summer camp. Directors who need to keep overtime in check can spread visits out over several months so staff time spent in any one week accrues as regular hours. One director arranges all visits during child care hours and shifts teachers' schedules to accommodate early morning and late afternoon appointments. This same director spends time in the classrooms herself to ensure coverage while teachers are out visiting when there are not enough substitutes to go around.

Build skills. Although there are plenty of caregivers who are natural home visitors, it is unrealistic for a program to expect first-time visits to be a complete success for everyone. Some teachers may need to go with a veteran mentor and observe—or be observed. A program could find that it takes a few years of home visiting before the activity becomes a strong asset to the program and all the elements are in place for every staff member a majority of the time. It takes a supportive director, a clear plan of action, a flexible team, and shared enthusiasm to bring everyone on board. As with anything new and challenging, understanding the value of home visiting and allowing for a period of experimentation go a long way toward making it succeed.

Dealing with the Challenging Side of Home Visits offers some additional strategies.

Dealing with the Challenging Side of Home Visits

Support. Home visiting works only if it has the full support of families, caregivers, and the director—especially the director. It helps if home visiting is program policy, so that all new staff and enrolling families know how important it is.

Collaboration. Visit in teams of two—maybe a pair of primary caregivers, a teacher and family support worker, or a caregiver and director. The team arrangement builds staff relationships as the pair make the rounds together.

Enthusiasm. Conveying an enthusiastic attitude is key to relationship building. One approach to inspire grumbling coworkers or convince a resistant director is for an individual caregiver to begin to make home visits on her own. As Tom Sawyer discovered about fence painting, when something starts to look like fun, naysayers are often lured into the project.

Reinforcement. Educating about the value of home visits and making annual visits a part of center policy can go a long way toward making successful visiting a reality.

Smart hiring. Directors can seek out caregivers who enjoy people of all ages, not just children. To succeed at home visiting, caregivers must appreciate adult relationships and value connections they make with parents. Selectivity in hiring helps eliminate internal sabotage of a home visiting program.

Relationships, the Heart of Quality Care

Strategy #4: Family participation

Open any book on early care and education and you will find a section dedicated to family participation or "parent involvement." It is an important feature of best practice and is widely encouraged in guidance and national standards. NAEYC (1997b) says that a developmentally appropriate program is one that makes whole families (even grandparents and siblings) welcome to visit the program and invites parents to participate in decisions about their children's care and education. The National Association for Family Child Care (2002) invites parents to become involved in program activities according to their interests and time availability. Parents are encouraged to become involved in all aspects of Early Head Start, including direct involvement in policy and program decisions that respond to parents' interests and needs (ACF 2003). All high-quality child care centers invite families to spend time in the classrooms, bring special snacks, go on field trips, add their cast-offs to the home living area, and share their skills and interests with the children.

In some programs parents are required to participate in the child's classroom a few hours a week. Most centers also have regular parent conferences, family newsletters, bulletin board displays, open house evenings, and regular events such as pizza night. Parents of infants and toddlers may be asked to take pictures, sew curtains, or wash blankets once a week. Families might be asked to help with fund-raising efforts, carnivals for the children, potluck dinners, and improvement projects such as building a toddler playground or painting a classroom. Some centers have parent advisory groups or a board position set aside for parents to help make policy and decisions. Notably, family involvement in program decision making is a hallmark of Head Start. The younger the child, the more likely it is that families will be interested—even eager—to be a part of center life in formal as well as informal ways. It is good to get parents started as soon as their children enter care. The number of ways to involve parents is limited only by the imagination and the enthusiasm of center staff.

Family participation brings parents into the center in the same way that home visits bring caregivers into the home, and with some of the same good results. When their families visit their center, children for a while have all their special adults together in the same place. Parents are able to observe caregivers interacting with their child, and it's the caregivers' turn to make parents feel welcome. In the best of circumstances, family participation builds relationships and a sense of community among all the adults. It makes home and center feel "seamless" for children and parents alike.

Benefits of family participation

For children. Children thrive when their parents participate in center activities—even if it is for just a short evening event. Their eyes light up, and they want to tell the world that this is a different and special moment—*"My mommy and daddy are here, and no one is rushing to say good-bye!"* Family participation bridges the gap between center and home. If parents see a caregiver using a familiar song to inspire cleanup, they are likely to try the same tactic at home. When there is connection and similarity between center and home, children feel secure within a circle of belonging. Life feels seamless, predictable, understandable.

For families. For most parents, feeling welcome in the center and spending time there with their children makes the time apart easier to bear. When families have regular opportunities to observe in the classroom, they don't have to wonder whether their children are noticed and treated with respect. The center's daily rhythm becomes familiar. Trust grows when parents see a caregiver remain calm when—all at the same time—Jerry throws a tantrum over a blue crayon, Charlene offers a messy hand to communicate her diarrhea, and Brianna and Ray fight over who made the blocks fall.

Family members who spend time in the center build relationships with staff and other parents. They feel less isolated and less guilty about leaving their children because they have become a part of the child care community themselves. Parents who serve on advisory committees, paint playground equipment, or participate in fund-raisers also refine skills useful in other parts of their lives. They develop a sense of pride in helping to make the center a better place for their own child and for everyone.

For caregivers. As with home visiting, caregivers get an opportunity to observe parent-child relationships in a nonthreatening context. Family participation offers regular opportunities for casual conversations and other adult interactions that increase continuity and consistency for the children, in turn making life easier for caregivers. Parents who spend time in the classroom or who do things to support center life after hours are more likely to appreciate their caregiver and look for other ways to help in the work he does each day. For example, a parent might wipe down the tables at the end of the day, read a story while the caregiver prepares snacks, or wash a child's hands—even if that child is not her own. These things build relationships and offer caregivers a little break from routine, which makes their job more satisfying.

Adult connections that develop make it even more natural to talk about problems and work on solutions together. For example, a caregiver became concerned about one mother's insistence on force-feeding her child. She explains,

> The little boy was healthy but slender. . . . She would force him to eat whether he was hungry or not, because she worried about his health. I felt that the child was thriving, so I suggested that she talk with a doctor about her concerns. I obtained information for her about child nutrition. It was hard for the mother to hear what I had to say, but she did because we had a close relationship. It would have been impossible to make an inroad otherwise.

We observed one preschool program in an affluent neighborhood in Southern California where family participation is producing dramatic results. Parents learn about children's development, discover new techniques for guiding behavior, and develop strong relationships with the caregivers. The adults have built a cohesive community that cares about the center, the children, and its members. In this climate of mutual respect, everyone thrives and caregivers remain on the job for decades.

For centers and directors. There are never enough hands or time or money to do everything that needs to be done in a child care center. Directors simply cannot do it all on their own—even with a superior staff and supportive board. Family participation helps many programs move beyond the basics by adding useful and personal touches from each parent's treasure trove of skills and joys. An artistic father creates an hall mural of amazing birds, fish, streams, and trees. A grandmother who is a printer produces professional-looking signs and newsletters for free or at cost. Other family members sign on as classroom helpers, plan celebrations, or find field-trip participants. Experienced directors know that family participation fosters a sense of ownership and pride in the center. This keeps parents coming back, supports staff, makes the center feel like a community, and, of course, surrounds the children with high-quality care.

Moving toward family participation

Inspiring busy parents to become involved in center life and stay involved over time is an ongoing challenge. Most center staff appreci-

"It was hard for the mother to hear what I had to say, but she did because we had a close relationship."

ate participation from family members, but counting on them to show up is a different matter. Open-house events are often well-attended, but everything else is unpredictable at best. Here are some strategies to make success of a family participation program more likely.

Authentic appreciation. Centers thriving on family contributions offer flexible, ongoing, choice-driven opportunities, something for everyone. They encourage parents to pick tasks that are easy to accomplish, and they enthusiastically appreciate whatever parents do, big or small. One professional mother who worked many hours a week wanted to be of help, but she didn't know what she could offer. She recalls,

> I went to my child's teacher and we finally agreed that what I could do is wash the cot sheets each week. She was thrilled. I have a machine at home, and it is no big deal to tote that little bundle each Friday. My older children help me fold them over the weekend—it's a family project and I like getting them involved with their little brother's life like this. On Monday I bring all these clean sheets as bright and happy gifts. It saves the teachers a bit of work and they really let me know it. Next year I will do two classrooms because I am pregnant and I'll have a new little one in the baby room. I like the idea that my child and his friends are sleeping on sheets I washed for them.

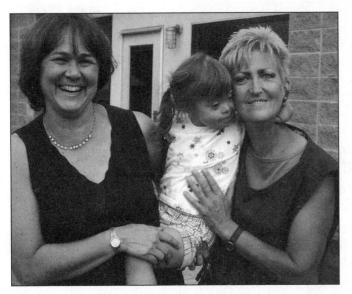

Most successful programs keep parent participation voluntary and try to come up with incentives to motivate involvement. Success depends a lot on relationships between staff and families. People by nature are more likely to do things— and go the extra mile—for those they think of as friends.

Mandatory participation. We visited two programs that rely on mandatory family participation to strengthen parent-caregiver relationships and get things done. One center has a large number of parents in transition from welfare to work; the second is a parent cooperative that serves professional families in an affluent urban neighborhood. In the program serving parents in transition, the parents can choose to volunteer for a few classroom hours or they can attend parenting classes. Many choose the classroom option because they enjoy being with their children and they learn from watching caregiver-child interactions. Says one mother,

> I learned a lot about discipline from working with Kathy. She rarely raised her voice and never made the kind of empty threats I do: "If you do that one more time, I'll … !" With her, the children knew there would be consequences to their actions.

In the parent co-op, family participation is tied to tuition discounts. Although every parent must contribute at least three hours of work per month, those who become more involved pay less than those who have more money than time to offer. Families choose the co-op because of the opportunity it offers to be a part of their children's daily lives. They also value the relationships they are able to develop with the other adults in this well-planned community. Mandatory participation sometimes makes it easier for parents to request time off at their workplaces or to find things to do after center hours.

Making parent participation mandatory is one sure way to get parents involved, but not every program has the inclination to do it or the luxury of insisting on it. Some center staff argue that it is too hard for parents to take time off from work to make participation mandatory. They try to make parents' lives easier by keeping requests for help to a minimum. In other cases, directors and other staff members don't want to "bother" parents with anything; as they see it, it is the center's job to cover the child's daily needs while parents concentrate on making a living.

Some parents are eager to participate in center life, but others wonder why they have to donate time and energy when they already pay fees. They don't realize how valuable the time spent at their children's center can be for everyone—including themselves. Some use the elementary-school model to defend their reasons for keeping out of the way. Others are new at parenting and still making the adjustment from life as a single or couple to one that revolves around a child.

Some staff resist the idea and even debate the value of parent participation. Some caregivers complain that parents are always "underfoot" and feel out of place in the center. The more interaction there is, caregivers argue, the more chance there is for parents to squabble with them over issues of control. To many, it seems easier to just leave well enough alone, keep families out of center business, and reduce the potential for conflict.

But as we have seen, family participation is well worth working out the challenges it might pose. The delight it brings to the children and its enhancements of program quality cannot be ignored. The question is not *whether* we should encourage family involvement but *how*.

Start small and build. A good first step is for staff and willing parents to develop a family participation *vision*. Create a series of action plans. Celebrate what's working and move slowly. Find ways to make the work pleasant and to show how much it helps the children and the program. Focus on creating community. A thriving community of participants encourages others to join in the fun. Get parents to recruit one another; assign participation partners to help a reserved parent or one with a particularly demanding schedule feel less stressed at the idea of volunteering.

Acknowledge caregivers. It also helps to recognize and appreciate teachers who welcome parents into their classrooms. Use staff meeting times to develop an appreciation for family participation programs and the role caregivers have in making parents feel welcome. Teach caregivers conflict-resolution skills, and discuss when and how to redirect *mis*-behaviors of parents who are trying to help out. Ask experienced caregivers to mentor their colleagues who are challenged or threatened by parents in the classroom.

The question is not *whether* we should encourage family involvement but *how*.

Value family participation. Look for ways to encourage parents to value time spent at their children's center. Collect stories that show other parents' pride and growth in this area. Publish the stories in the program newsletter—the mother who's learning more-effective guidance methods, the grandfather who enjoys taking pictures of the children, the father who likes to share storybooks. Be sure to emphasize the concepts of building community and developing seamless care between home and center.

Watch parents and get to know them. Reach out. Offer diverse possibilities for their becoming involved. Base invitations to participate on parents' observed strengths. Few human beings can resist a request that begins, "I have been watching you and I can see you are wonderful at . . ." or "I hear you know how to. . . ." People generally enjoy doing what they do well, and they will contribute that skill if they can find the time.

Don't shame families into participating. Think in terms of positive reinforcement and motivation strategies. For example, in the monthly newsletter or on a bulletin board thank those families who are already involved. You can also list opportunities that read like help-wanted ads. Make sure there are options that require only a short amount of time. Some parents feel less stressed if they can choose something just once in a while instead of making a regular monthly commitment. Offer regular chances to change or renew commitments, rather than waiting until you see signs of flagging interest or energy.

Consider making family participation mandatory. You may want to make some kind of commitment a part of the intake process. If participation is promoted from the beginning, parents who are unwilling or unable to become involved will weed themselves out of the center. The energy and quality that family involvement adds to a program outweigh any challenges it can bring. Programs should hire caregivers who like and value adults as well as children. Emphasize that in child care, working well with adults is part of the job, that caregivers who thrive are the ones who enjoy being with people of all ages.

Strategy #5: Family-supportive care

The goal of family-supportive child care is to go beyond daily services that provide direct support to the child, such as feeding, napping, and managing children's behavior. By creating networks of social support, family-supportive care strengthens parents' self-esteem and breaks down barriers that separate caregivers and parents. Also called "family-centered care," such programs respond to family needs by offering such things as parenting classes, dinners-to-go, auto mechanics classes, dry-cleaning pickup, even an occasional night out while children are cared for at the center, for nominal fees. Like the family model, family-supportive care is based in the idea that the core of quality lies in encouraging adult relationships.

Family-supportive child care is part of a broad national movement based on best-practice models developed by Head Start, the nonprofit Parent Services Project (PSP), and other family-friendly child care programs (Pope & Seiderman 2000–01).

In Head Start a family caseworker meets with each family individually to plan for the needs of child and parents. Using her familiarity with all the families, the caseworker recommends center-wide programs and activities to serve families who share similar challenges or interests. Like other family-centered programs, Head Start programs also form parent advisory groups to plan supportive family activities. They foster good rapport between parents and caregivers to work together for the sake of the children. Head Start caregivers often see

> Programs should hire caregivers who like and value adults as well as children.

PSP: One Model of Family-Supportive Care

"If your work is children, then your work is families," says Ethel Seiderman, founder and executive director of the Parent Services Project (PSP). This innovative, San Francisco Bay–area nonprofit organization has been focusing on the importance of adult relationships in child care settings since the late 1970s. Its family-supportive strategies are now used by more than 700 child care programs, serving more than 25,000 families in eight states with training and technical assistance.

PSP promotes family support values and practices, which guide programs to build, carry, and promote reciprocal relationships among the adults in the early childhood community. In addition to a strong focus on relationship building, families and program staff at a site develop activities and resource links that meet the unique needs and interests of those families. That makes every site seem very different—at least on the surface. As Seiderman points out, "It looks simple, but instead it is simply profound."

PSP's underlying principles are the bedrock of its work:
• Partnership
• Share Power
• Family Strengths
• Cultural Competence
• Family Driven
• Social Support
• Hope and Joy

The PSP approach is grounded in mutual respect, parent leadership, staff-parent partnerships, and family empowerment. Training is based on relationships, shared stories, and the importance of supporting families in ways that allow them to support the lives of their children. Seiderman offers several lessons that PSP has learned about creating family-supportive care:

Start with who shows up. Don't worry about numbers. Keep offering choices that encourage attendance, but don't mandate it. Let relationships grow naturally, and trust in the power of the group to pull other people into the circle.

Acknowledge that relationship building is challenging, time-consuming work— especially at first. Expect some resistance. Persuade; don't push. Allow adults to open

themselves as extensions of the family unit, like a grandmother or uncle. They suggest community opportunities and resources to support parents in rearing children, improving job skills, and meeting other adult challenges.

California-based PSP has spent decades researching, implementing, and promoting the notion that providing support to parents strengthens the entire family. With PSP's training and technical assistance, a center might help family members develop parenting and job skills or learn first aid. Parents gain a growing sense of competency as they begin to realize they are the most important people in their child's life. Those who become involved acquire leadership skills by making and tailoring programs to meet participating families' needs. Together, adults and children alike are invited to enjoy family and community activities that are particularly designed to build relation-

up to one another in their own ways and on their own timetables. Says Seiderman, "Own any problems as soon as they arise. Relate to such challenges by acknowledging their presence. Leave room for the group to see what's needed to work through issues and to problem solve with the people involved." Place value on relationships as a quality component of early care.

Hire a "family support coordinator" to work with families to organize and energize services, activities, and meetings. A center of 100 families would need a full-time person; the entire program might cost $300-400 per family per year (just $7 extra per family per week). A smaller center could create a part-time support position. It is also possible for a staff member to assume this role and be compensated—if it is a match.

Establish a "family leadership group" and encourage those parents whom staff see as particularly thoughtful and constructive to join. This group advises and sets goals for PSP relationship building. It taps into the interests and needs of all parents, reflecting this in program planning, thus this becomes part of the site culture.

Choose a "parent leadership liaison" from the family leadership group. This person might be paid a small stipend to work with the family support coordinator to align efforts between the parent group and the center staff and develop a vibrant, effective family-centered program.

Focus and build on strengths of the group. See the potential offered by strong, sustaining relationships in child care centers, and develop trust among families and staff members over time.

View services as a vehicle to create community. Community empowers people and allows them to find strengths in themselves they might not even know they have.

For more about PSP, visit its Web site at www.parentservices.org. Or contact Parent Services Project, Inc., 79 Belvedere St., Suite 101, San Rafael, CA 94901. Email: family@ parentservices.org. Ph: 415-454-1870. Fax: 415-454-1752.

ships among the adults. **PSP: One Model of Family-Supportive Care** offers more details about the approach.

Benefits of family-supportive care

For children. In family-supportive child care centers, regular gatherings planned for adults encircle children in an ongoing community of family members and center staff that operates much like an extended family or a close-knit congregation. Adults naturally begin to help one another in friendly, human ways. After-hours activities in the center, along with time spent away together, help relationships grow. Adult interactions are mimicked in children's behavior toward others and become a model for future use as well. Center-planned family supports, such as reasonably priced meals made by the cook for

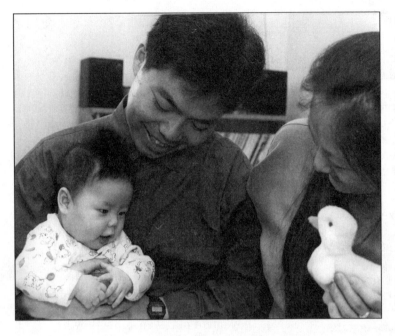

afternoon pickup, give everyone time to dawdle at the center together. The usual supper rush is traded for a relaxed mealtime, during which 2-year-old Bobby elicits delight and laughter rather than impatience from Mom and Dad for singing *Twinkle Star* over and over and *over* again.

As early care and education professionals, we know that children's self-esteem and confidence are linked to the level of parent involvement and to care that is relatively similar whether children are at home or at the center. When a program adds a menu of adult-focused participation opportunities, involvement of one kind or another usually follows, and children thrive. In family-supportive centers shared learning between parents and caregivers also means higher quality care for children both at home and at the center. As bonds are forged, the adults' self-esteem grows in both "homes," and their conversations weave a seamless world that even babies can sense.

For families. In earlier generations, family support was the domain of one's biological family. Brothers, sisters, aunts, uncles, grandparents could often be called upon to run errands, watch children, offer wisdom and advice, and help in emergencies. Today many families are spread out and spread thin. Relatives frequently are too far away or too busy themselves to be of much help. The family-supportive approach recognizes this reality and encourages centers to consider family needs in program planning to reduce parents' isolation and create a caring community.

Adult relationships in family-supportive centers evolve naturally, like those in a neighborhood. If a parent misses seeing her child's caregiver Friday at pick-up time, thanks to center-organized events she may have another chance at that evening' ball game or on Saturday's trip to the outlet store. The center becomes a place for the adults to gather, exchange ideas, and explore joys and concerns with those they

Relationships, the Heart of Quality Care

have grown to care for and who care about them. It is a place to come "home" to after a long day at work.

For caregivers. Family-supportive care makes life easier for caregivers in the long run, even given their time spent on that extra layer of support, because caregivers, and usually their families, are included in the center-based community that results. The enlivening community spirit invites adults to bond, to chat about life, to get to know one another in authentic ways. In one family-supportive center we observed, it was hard to tell caregiver from parent at pick-up time. The adults were bouncing in and out of conversations, smiling, laughing, taking their time. No one was in a hurry to go home; they *were* home. The day we were there, "carry-home" suppers were ready and waiting for everyone to take along, so staff as well as parents felt the luxury of time to hang out. With this kind of community as the reward, it is easy to see why busy caregivers are happy to make the extra effort.

When adults relax together they find the attitude and time they need to build trust with one another. In such an environment, information may pop up during informal exchanges that a caregiver otherwise might never have thought to ask about. For example, during a bus ride to an outing, one mother volunteered to her caregiver that she was caught in an uncomfortable situation: her husband and her mother couldn't stand each other. "I hate being in the middle," she confided. "I love them both. I don't know why they can't get along. . . . I am afraid Emily can't help but hear, and it is very confusing to her." The caregiver wondered whether the tension might explain Emily's occasional acting out, and he felt comfortable asking the mother about it. Their conversation was easy, natural, and the problem was solved before it got out of hand . . . the way it's done between friends.

Caregivers who become close to parents through shared experiences often find themselves supported during their own challenges. One caregiver says she was able to survive the first few months of divorce because of the kind and sensitive conversations she had with parents. In a mutually trusting relationship, the value of sharing lives works both ways, like family at its best.

For directors and centers. Directors in family-supportive centers are usually clear about all the benefits described above; they talk about them with big smiles on their faces. One director took us on a grand tour, pointing out all the things the families decided on to make the center's classrooms more homey. After their first meeting as a family support advisory board, parents installed bright curtains, hanging plants, fish tanks, soft pillows for the book area—even a twin bed in one of the classrooms—so the center would look less "institutional."

Shared projects are one of the many ways that families and staff build their relationships. These parents took a lot of pride in their improvements, and the director was particularly pleased to say that they regularly invite the caregivers in on the fun. One Saturday several parents went to a movie, leaving the children at the center with caregivers who had volunteered to be the parents' paid babysitters. They had such a good time, they included the caregivers the next time, leaving parent volunteers with the children. It makes any director's job easier when she works with an eager and thoughtful community of adults like this one.

Moving toward family-supportive care

From its beginning in the 1960s, Head Start has respected individual family values as a core principle of each program. Now, along with Early Head Start, it recognizes that values differ from family to family and from community to community and that children should be raised within the context of their home values to encourage a seamless experience in their young years. That many Head Start teachers are parents themselves and all are part of the community continues to be a critical factor in the success of this long-running family-friendly model.

A testimonial from a PSP brochure (2001) brings the need for family-supportive programs into brilliant clarity:

> I used to think my job was just about caring for the children. But the longer I worked, the more I realized that each child comes to you with a family and [each child goes] home to a family. In the life of a child, child care providers and schools may change, but the family is the constant. If you care about the child, you have to care about the family.
>
> When it's about what's best for the children, there's no room for "us and them." Children need all of us working together on their behalf. They need everyone's strengths. They need to know that we are connected to one another. Family support is about building caring and respectful relationships all around our children. Children need that. Parents need that. Caregivers need that too.

Family-supportive child care rests on the philosophy that every parent is a decision maker. Each parent knows his or her own needs, knows which activities are helpful or of interest, and has something to contribute to the group. Family-supportive programs create conditions that enable families, caregivers, and directors to share their own interests and build on their own strengths.

At the Community Lab School for Family Supportive Child Care, in Fort Worth, Texas, onsite services for harried parents include exercise classes, one-day dry cleaning, snack sales, take-home meals, stamp sales, and a mailbox (Pope & Seiderman 2000-01). In Georgia a group of providers and families share field trips, picnics, and Thanksgiving dinners. Their annual fashion show generates funds for each year's plans. At All My Heart Educational Center, in Cleveland, Ohio, families and caregivers go on field trips to the airport and the natural history museum. On the bus on the way to a baseball game (free tickets for families and caregivers!), a coach talks about helping children choose appropriate sports activities. Such family-supportive programs know that joy and fun are essential to communication and family well-being and for strengthening the pathways of excellence in care. It's an after-hours club that everyone is welcome to join.

One thing leads to another as adults become more comfortable with one another. They begin to plan information-sharing or skill-building activities, such as programs on home financing, drug and alcohol abuse, car repair, women's health, managing stress, good parenting, even scrapbooking. They come together on social occasions, such as potlucks and excursions, and over committee work or fundraising efforts. Participation certainly is not mandatory, but when adults attend, they find they have much in common.

These programs are successful because families are in charge. When they decide for themselves that they want classes in guidance or cooking Thai food and they search out a speaker or discussion leader

---

Getting Started with Family-Supportive Child Care

• Greet families warmly at drop-off and pick-up times.

• Show interest in what's going on with families.

• Plan informal activities such as picnics or trips to the zoo that allow families to have fun with their children while getting to know staff.

• Schedule some adults-only events and arrange for child care. Families and staff benefit from occasions that allow bonds to form outside of the child care arrangement.

• Let families know their opinions count. Invite their suggestions—one on one or through a bulletin board or a suggestion box.

• Publicize the suggestions families make; publicize your responses.

• Post announcements of social events; post sign-up sheets for group participation.

• Cook and package take-out meals that families (caregivers too) can order. Because the adults won't have to rush home to fix dinner, they can relax and chat together for a while at the center.

• Create a parent-staff council to plan training events and engage speakers.

on that topic and help set the price for tickets, they are also more likely to attend. Simply stated, in family-supportive child care, parents, directors, and caregivers share adult interests and friendships blossom. Adult connection and support, which might seem like extras, become the cornerstone of seamless high-quality care for children.

The box **Getting Started with Family-Supportive Child Care** (on page 169) offers some simple ideas. Barriers to family-supportive care typically take two forms. First is the assumption that the program knows what is best for families, better than the families know themselves. A second is to see the family-supportive approach as a big bother.

"We know what you need." Some "parent involvement" programs are arranged by well-intentioned staff members who believe they already know what families need without asking. They plan services and activities without collecting parent input and then wonder why no one shows up. They dismiss the discomfort many adults have with a formal school setting, never connecting poor attendance at center functions with parents' own school memories of feeling inferior or lazy or stupid. Staff in such programs may even see parents as adversaries and focus on the "problems" families create for them day after day. When that focus guides decision making, programs host classes or support groups with the aim of changing parents' behavior or "fixing" their way of raising children. The attitude is *"it's for their own good."* When a program thinks this way, parents resist rather than welcome the "support." In family-supportive child care, no one feels superior.

"It's too much trouble." Some detractors of family-supportive care question the value of putting so much time and energy into the *adults* when, in their view, the proper job of a caregiver is to care for *children*. Staff in such programs complain, "We don't have time for all this foolishness, and parents don't want to spend their time off hanging around here. Besides, they need to be home with their children." In such an environment relationships are the furthest thing from staff members' minds, and families respond in kind. Using the business and school models as their reference, the adults keep their interactions limited and hierarchical, the way they typically do in those settings.

"And *who* is going to pay for all this?" Money can seem like a barrier to offering family-supportive activities. However, part of the concept, especially as developed by PSP, is to include financial considerations in the planning process. In some cases the committee may decide to arrange for services that parents would pay for elsewhere, and offer the services at a fair price. Parents might even agree to pay *more* for the convenience of having dry cleaning or mailing services all in one convenient place. In other cases a group might decide to raise funds to cover the costs of a bus trip or special speaker in order to offer the event to the community for free. Usually, those involved discover that planning for costs and meeting goals as a *team* is part of the community-building fun.

A community of caring adults

Connections among adults who share the care of young children are strengthened by the strategies described here—using the family model to shape workplace policies, community building, home visits, parent participation, family-supportive care. Relationships built by these connections encircle children with a community of people who care about one another as well as them. The result is high-quality care.

Sometimes all it takes to start on that path to community is a little encouragement. Encouragement can mean a center putting new family-friendly policies in place. Or deciding that adults should meet together regularly on each another's turf. In some cases it means giving adults permission to become close even if there is a contract with a fee for service. Yes, fires must be put out now and then; relationships can become messy, and feelings can get hurt. But adults who develop trusting connections work together more willingly to meet children's needs than do those who keep their distance. The realization that they belong to a caring community increases the depth and longevity of their commitment, much to the benefit of the children. We cannot ignore this fact: Authentic, nurturing community benefits everyone—today and long after the child care years are over, when it is our children's turn to live what they learned in their earliest years.

◆   ◆   ◆

In these last three chapters we explored some of the best strategies we know for achieving child-centered, relationship-based child care communities. Our last chapter, **Conversations of the Heart,** is our call to action. It poses questions for you to ponder individually and with other adults in your child care world. The chapter offers a starting point from which to validate your strengths and explore areas in need of further growth. We challenge you to bring your program to the heights of relationship-based care that high-quality family child care homes and a growing number of enlightened centers, including those featured in this book, are already offering.

Join us on the journey to excellence. Make your center a model of child-centered, relationship-based care. Become an authentic community in which caring is the goal and everyone thrives.

The next steps are yours.

6

Conversations of the Heart: Next Steps

Although we have described the strengths of family child care and promoted the family model as important examples of relationship-based care for centers, we know that no care setting for children during their early years is "perfect"—not even their home. Each setting—the home, family child care, the child care center—has its assets and challenges; each has something to teach the field of early care and education. To talk about the *best* setting for young children is both fruitless and alienating. Instead we must always return to the question that should inspire our work: What do children need to *thrive*—no matter where they spend their days?

We know that children thrive when they are surrounded with love. We know that all functional families and communities feature meaningful adult relationships and encircle their children with people who care. It is time to apply the lessons of success that home and family offer us for rearing children to be competent, emotionally healthy adults. If we are to create centers and systems that truly meet the needs of young children, early care and education professionals must go beyond typical thinking. We must challenge ourselves—both individually and as a profession—with new questions.

We ourselves have begun by talking explicitly in workshops with caregivers and directors about the ways they meet children's needs for bonding and attachment. We ask our colleagues about their feelings for children in care: "Are you comfortable when you form emotional attachments to a child? How do the parents feel?" And we talk about center policies: "Which ones strengthen relationships between families and caregivers? Do any weaken or undermine that connection?"

Discussions reveal a continuum of possibilities. For example, some centers permit caregivers to take on extra hours of care for families on weekends; some forbid off-site babysitting; other programs do not forbid it but don't want to know when it happens either. Centers have different ways of welcoming new families to their programs: In some, the director meets with enrolling parents; in others, the director and caregivers talk privately with the parents; in still others, caregivers make a visit to the family's home.

Believing that awareness is the first step toward change, our discussions are meant to be nonthreatening, giving participants a chance to consider their own beliefs and listen to their coworkers' points of view. Self-reflectiveness is the goal. Staff members and centers must consider their own unique circumstances. But there is a bottom line that cannot be ignored—some policies *strengthen* parent-caregiver relationships, and some *weaken* them. Awareness is the first step toward change.

Discussions can have a ripple effect. A director with 20 years of experience describes the impact a workshop had on her and her staff:

> Most of my staff has been with me for more than 10 years, and they know about the importance of relationships. But it's new to think that relationships are priority. . . . It's got us thinking again.

Our goal with this final chapter is to magnify the ripple effect into a force for change. We encourage you to take next steps: To enter into conversations about relationships—*the heart of quality care.* To set up dialogues between and among parents and staff members in your own child care setting. To reflect on what you are doing—as individuals and as groups of coworkers—about meeting children's needs for bonding and attachment, especially those of infants, toddlers, and children with special needs. Could you do more? Do your relationships with families go beyond cordial formality to real connection, caring, and trust? Do your program policies support the kinds of adult relationships that underlie quality care, or do they get in the way?

Start the conversation—formally at workshops, conferences, and staff meetings or informally during the course of a day. By talking together, you will discover what it will take to carry your program and the field of early care and education forward. We are all learning as we go, so free yourself from any fear that there are right or wrong answers.

Here are some discussion questions we have found useful to help you get started.

Let's talk about attitudes and perceptions

Love and attachment

- Do you feel you know enough about attachment, or should you learn more about its importance for young children?

- Are you comfortable when you become attached to children in your care? Do you worry about having favorites?

- Are you comfortable when children bond with you? Do you ever feel embarrassed?

- Are you comfortable when you see emotional attachment between another caregiver and a child? Are some caregiver-child attachments unhealthy? Why?

- Do you ever sense that you or your coworkers compete with parents for their children's affection?

- Do parents at your center value attachments that form between caregivers and children? Are parents ever fearful or threatened by such attachments? What do you do to reassure them that attachments are necessary and good for children?

- Would families at your center benefit from learning more about the importance of attachment in their children's lives?

Formality and friendship

- How do you define professionalism in relating to families and other staff? Do your coworkers agree with that definition?

- How close do you think caregivers should get to parents? When do parent-caregiver relationships become too close?

- Are you able to form close, caring relationships with all the parents of the children in your care? Do you need any help in strengthening those relationships?

- What do you do to maintain fairness and manage adult expectations among families when certain caregivers and parents become friends?

Families

- How much do you know about the other important people in the lives of the children you care for?

- Are you comfortable talking with children about missing their mommy or daddy? Do you hesitate during the day to refer to the parent because you don't want to make the child cry?

- Do you see situations in which children have to deal with major inconsistencies in their home versus center care or with tension

> By talking together, you will discover what it will take to carry your program and the field of early care and education forward.

between their parents and their caregiver? Are there any other steps you can take to ensure that children receive seamless care?

■ Do you ever fear knowing too much about a family's circumstances or not knowing what to do with information? Would it be helpful to talk with a professional who studies families who are dysfunctional or in crisis?

Let's talk about center policies

■ How do your center's policies strengthen relationships between adults? between adults and children?

■ Do any of your center's policies weaken or undermine relationships? Which policies?

■ What do you need to know to establish policies that are more supportive of adult relationships?

■ Do your center's policies support caring connections with parents that go beyond formal cordiality?

■ Do its policies limit staff relationships with families? Why? For instance, how does the program view out-of-center parent-caregiver contact? caregivers babysitting for families after hours?

■ What do you need to know before you can introduce primary caregiving and continuity of care into your infant/toddler program?

■ Does your center have policies on gradual transitioning of infants and toddlers? What do you need to know to make transitions easier for families and children?

■ Do you need to make changes in staff scheduling so relationship priorities are put first? For instance, is there frequent contact between parents and their child's primary caregiver?

Let's talk about individual initiatives

■ What insights have led you and your coworkers to strengthen relationships with one another? with parents?

■ What steps have you or your coworkers taken to strengthen relationships at your center?

■ Does your center have a way to acknowledge or celebrate these steps?

■ Should your center do more to acknowledge and support caregivers who act on their own initiative to strengthen relationships? What should it do?

Let's talk about indicators of quality

National standards acknowledge adult relationships as indicators of quality child care, but most assessment tools lack criteria for evaluating the strength of those relationships. Let's discuss some possible criteria.

- Is a primary caregiver assigned to each infant and toddler? Do the parents know about their child's assignment? Does the primary caregiver focus mainly on her own group for nurturing routines such as meals, naps, diaper changes, and small-group gatherings? Do children call her by name?

- How often do primary caregivers and parents interact: daily? weekly? only sporadically?

- Does the center support continuity of care? How? How long is continuity ensured for infants and toddlers?

- Do caregivers keep in touch with children and families after the caregiving period ends?

- Do caregivers talk during the day to the children about their mommies and daddies?

- How do caregivers support children in the context of the family? For instance, are children permitted to bring things from home? Are photos of family members on hand for the children to look at? Can children call their parents during the day? What other means are used to support children's relationships with their families?

- Does the center have access to outside professionals to help staff understand families who are in trouble or in crisis?

Let's talk about family perspectives

- Do families see the importance of their relationship with their child's caregiver?

- Do families appreciate their child's caregiver, or do they need ideas about ways to show that appreciation—for instance, thank yous, offers of help, or gestures such as a note or flowers?

- Do families know that it's normal for children to come to love their caregiver, and that such attachment is good for their child's development?

- Do families understand that children are capable of loving more than one person, and that loving a caregiver doesn't undermine a child's love for a parent?

- Is anyone talking to families about the importance of creating a close connection with their child's caregiver that is strong enough to sustain them through conflict?
- Are parents encouraged to work to overcome differences with their child's caregiver, especially when the child and caregiver have bonded?
- Is anyone conducting home visits?
- Is family participation a shared value and goal among center staff? among parents?
- What is being done to increase family-supportive care?
- Are families and staff members sharing life and joy with one another?
- Does your center "feel like home"?
- Is relationship and community building a center-wide goal?

The journey of a thousand miles begins with a single step.
—Japanese proverb

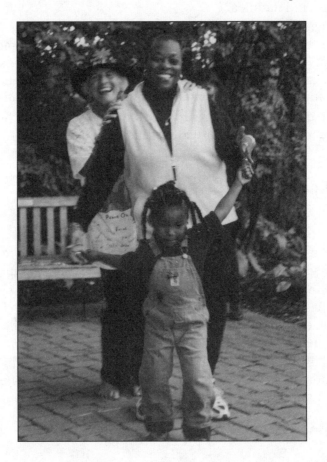

Relationships, the Heart of Quality Care

Resources

Publications, national standards, and assessment scales

Administration for Children and Families (ACF). 2003, June. *Program performance measures for Head Start programs serving infants and toddlers.* Washington, DC: U.S. Department of Health and Human Services. Available online at www.acf.hhs.gov/programs/core/ongoing_research/ehs/prgm_perf_measures/perf_meas_4pg.html.

Ainsworth, M., & S. Bell. 1974. Mother-infant interaction and the development of competence. In *The growth of competence,* eds. K. Connolly & J. Bruner, 97–118. New York: Academic Press.

Albrecht, K., M. Banks, G. Calhoun, L. Dziadul, C. Gwinn, B. Herrington, B. Kerr, M. Mizukami, A. Morris, C. Peterson, & R.R. Summers. 2000. Keeping children and caregivers together: The good, the bad, and the wonderful. *Child Care Information Exchange* (November/December): 24–28.

Albrecht, K., L. Dziadul, C. Gwinn, & B. Herrington. 2001. Keeping children and caregivers together (part 2): The good, the bad, and the wonderful. *Child Care Information Exchange* (January/February): 90–94.

American Academy of Pediatrics (AAP), American Public Health Association (APHA), & National Resource Center for Health and Safety in Child Care (NRCHSCC). 2002. *Caring for our children—National health and safety performance standards: Guidelines for out-of-home child care.* 2d ed. Elk Grove Village, IL: American Academy of Pediatrics; Washington, DC: American Public Health Association; and Aurora, CO: National Resource Center for Health and Safety in Child Care. Available online at http://nrc.uchsc.edu/.

Arend, R., F.L. Gove, & L.A. Sroufe. 1979. Continuity of individual adaptation from infancy to kindergarten: A predictive study of ego resiliency and curiosity in preschoolers. *Child Development* 50 (4): 950–59.

Baker, A.C., & L.A. Manfredi/Petitt. 1998. *Circle of love: Relationships between parents, children, and caregivers in family child care.* St. Paul, MN: Redleaf.

Bales, D., & C. Campbell, eds. 2002, Spring. *Better brains for babies.* 2d ed. Trainer's manual. Athens, GA: University of Georgia/College of Family and Consumer Sciences and Georgia State University/School of Nursing. [More at www.bbbgeorgia.org]

Barnard, K., & G. Sumner. 1996. *Keys to caregiving.* Seattle: NCAST, University of Washington.

Barnas, M.V., & E.M. Cummings. 1997. Caregiver stability and toddlers' attachment-related behaviors towards caregivers in day care. *Infant Behavior and Development* 17: 171–77.

Bennett-Goleman, T. 2001. *Emotional alchemy: How the mind can heal the heart.* New York: Harmony.

Bernhardt, J.L. 2000, March. A primary caregiving system for infants and toddlers: Best for everyone involved. *Young Children* 55 (2): 74–80.

Bertacchi, V. 1996. Relationship-based organizations. *Zero to Three* 17 (2): 1–7.

Bloom, P.J. 1997. *A great place to work: Improving conditions for staff in young children's programs.* Rev. ed. Washington, DC: NAEYC.

Bloom, P.J., P. Eisenberg, & E. Eisenberg. 2003. Reshaping early childhood programs to be more family responsive. *America's Family Support Magazine* (Spring/Summer): 36–38.

Bove, C. 1999, March. *L'inserimento del bambino al nido* (Welcoming the child into child care): Perspectives from Italy. *Young Children* 54 (2): 32–34.

Bowlby, J. 1969. *Attachment*. Vol. 1 of *Attachment and loss*. New York: Basic.

Bowlby, J. 1973. *Separation: Anxiety and anger*. Vol. 2 of *Attachment and loss*. New York: Basic.

Bowlby, J. 1980. *Loss: Sadness and depression*. Vol. 3 of *Attachment and loss*. New York: Basic.

Brand, S. 1996, January. Making parent involvement a reality: Helping teachers develop partnerships with parents. *Young Children* 51 (2): 76–81.

Brazelton, T.B. 1990a. *Families: Crisis and caring*. New York: Ballantine.

Brazelton, T.B. 1990b. *Touchpoints: Your child's emotional and behavioral development*. Reading, MA: Addison-Wesley.

Brazelton, T.B. 1992. *Touchpoints: Your child's emotional and behavioral development: Birth–3: The essential reference for the early years*. Cambridge, MA: Perseus.

Brazelton, T.B., & B.G. Cramer. 1990. *The earliest relationship: Parents, infants, and the drama of early attachment*. Reading, MA: Addison-Wesley.

Brazelton, T.B., & S.I. Greenspan. 2000. *The irreducible needs of children: What every child must have to grow, learn, and flourish*. Cambridge, MA: Perseus.

Brazelton, T.B., & J.D. Sparrow. 2002. *Touchpoints three to six: Your child's emotional and behavioral development*. Cambridge, MA: Perseus.

Bredekamp, S., & C. Copple, eds. 1997. *Developmentally appropriate practice in early childhood programs*. Rev. ed. Washington, DC: NAEYC.

Bronfenbrenner, U. 1991, Winter/Spring. What do families do? *Family Affairs* 4 (1–2): 1–6.

Buber, M. 1965. *Between man and man*. New York: Macmillan.

Buffin, L. 2001. Relationships in child care settings: Becoming fully human (or what matters most). *Child Care Information Exchange* (January/February): 16–18.

Buscaglia, L. 1982. *Living, loving, and learning*. New York: Fawcett Columbine.

Carlson, V.J., & R.L. Harwood. 1999–2000. Understanding and negotiating cultural differences concerning early developmental competence: The six raisin solution. *Zero to Three* 20 (3): 19–23.

Carter, M. 2001. Indicators of effective teamwork. *Child Care Information Exchange* (January/February): 68–71.

Cassidy, J., & P.R. Shaver, eds. 1999. *Handbook of attachment: Theory, research, and clinical applications*. New York: Guilford.

Center for the Child Care Workforce. 2001, April. *Then and now: Changes in child care staffing 1994–2000*. Washington, DC: Author.

Children's Foundation. 2003. *2003 Child care licensing study*. Washington, DC: Author.

Children's Institute International. 1999. Early childhood and brain development. *CII Forum* (Winter): 1–2.

Chodron, P. 1996. *Awakening loving-kindness*. Boston: Shambhala.

Chodron, P. 2001. *The places that scare you: A guide to fearlessness in difficult times*. Boston: Shambhala.

Cleary, T. 1999. *The pocket Zen reader*. Boston: Shambhala.

Copple, C., ed. 2003. *A world of difference: Readings on teaching young children in a diverse society*. Washington, DC: NAEYC.

Curran, D. 1983. *Traits of a happy family*. New York: Harper & Row.

Daniel, J.E. 1998, November. A modern mother's place is wherever her children are: Facilitating infant and toddler mothers' transitions in child care. *Young Children* 53 (6): 4–12.

DeLoache, J., & A. Gottlieb. 2000. *A world of babies: Imagined childcare guides for seven societies*. Cambridge, UK: Cambridge University Press.

Derman-Sparks, L., and the A.B.C. Task Force. 1989. *Anti-bias curriculum: Tools for empowering young children*. Washington, DC: NAEYC.

Diffily, D. 2001. Family meetings: Teachers and families build relationships. *Dimensions of Early Childhood* (Summer): 5–9.

DiNatale, L. 2002, September. Developing high-quality family involvement programs in early childhood settings. *Young Children* 57 (5): 90–95.

Dodge, D.T., & C. Heroman. 1999. *Building your baby's brain: A parent's guide to the first five years*. Washington, DC: Teaching Strategies.

Dombro, A.L., & P. Bryan. 1991. *Sharing the caring: How to find the right child care and make it work for you and your child*. New York: Simon and Schuster.

Dombro, A.L., J. Colker, & D.T. Dodge. 1999. *The creative curriculum for infants and toddlers*. Rev. ed. Washington, DC: Teaching Strategies.

Education Commission of the States (ECS). 2001. *Starting early, starting now: A policy maker's guide to early care and education and school success*. Denver: Author.

Edwards, C.P., L. Gandini, & G. Forman, eds. 1998. *The hundred languages of children: The Reggio Emilia approach—Advanced reflections*. 2d ed. Greenwich, CT: Ablex.

Edwards, C.P., & H. Raikes. 2002, July. Extending the dance: Relationship-based approaches to infant/toddler care and education. *Young Children* 57 (4): 10–17.

Ehrensaft, D. 1987. *Parenting together*. New York: Free Press.

Ehrensaft, D. 1997. *Spoiling childhood. How well-meaning parents are giving children too much—But not what they need*. New York: Guilford.

Elicker, J., I.C. Noppe, & L.D. Noppe. 1996. Parent-Caregiver Relationship Scale.

Elkind, D. 1994. *Ties that stress: The new family imbalance*. Cambridge, MA: Harvard University Press.

Emde, R.N., T.L. Mann, & J. Bertacchi. 2001, August/September. Organizational environments that support mental health. *Zero to Three* 22 (1): 67–69.

Erickson, M.F., J. Korfmacher, & B. Egeland. 1992. Attachments past and present: Implications for therapeutic intervention with mother-infant dyads. *Development and Psychopathology* 4: 495–507.

Erikson, E.H. 1950. *Childhood and society*. New York: Norton.

Fox, I. 1996. *Being there: The benefits of a stay-at-home parent*. New York: Barron's.

Fraiberg, S. 1959. *The magic years*. New York: Scribner's.

Fraiberg, S. 1977. *Every child's birthright: In defense of mothering*. New York: Basic.

Furman, E., ed. 1986. *What nursery school teachers ask us about: Psychoanalytic consultations in preschool*. Madison, CT: International Universities Press.

Furman, E. 1987. *Helping young children grow: "I never knew parents did so much."* Madison, CT: International Universities Press.

Furman, E. 1993. *Toddlers and their mothers. Abridged version for parents and educators*. Madison, CT: International Universities Press.

Furman, E., ed. 1995. *Preschoolers: Questions and answers. Psychoanalytic consultations with parents, teachers, and caregivers*. Madison, CT: International Universities Press.

Galinsky, E. 1988, March. Parents and teacher-caregivers: Sources of tension, sources of support. *Young Children* 43 (3): 4–12.

Gandini, L., & C.P. Edwards. 2001. *Bambini: The Italian approach to infant/toddler care*. New York: Teachers College Press.

Garbarino, J. 2001. Power struggles: Early experiences matter. *Child Care Information Exchange* (January/February): 55–58.

Goldstein, L. 1997. *Teaching with love: A feminist approach to early childhood education*. New York: Peter Lang.

Goncu, A., & E. Klein, eds. 2001. *Children in play, story, and school*. New York: Greenwood.

Gonzalez-Mena, J. 1997. *Multicultural issues in child care*. 2d ed. Mountainview, CA: Mayfield Publishing.

Gonzalez-Mena, J. 2001. Personal power: Creating new realities. *Child Care Information Exchange* (January/February): 59–62.

Gonzalez-Mena, J., & A. Stonehouse. 2003. High-maintenance parent or parent partner? Working with a parent's concern. *Child Care Information Exchange.* (July/August): 16–18.

Granju, K.A., & B. Kennedy. 1999. *Attachment parenting: Instinctive care for your baby and young child.* New York: Pocket Books.

Greenberg, P. 1991. *Character development: Encouraging self-esteem and self-discipline in infants, toddlers, and two-year-olds.* Washington, DC: NAEYC.

Greenman, J. 1988. *Caring spaces, learning places: Children's environments that work.* Redmond, WA: Exchange Press.

Greenman, J. 1996. *Prime times: A handbook for excellence in infant and toddler programs.* St. Paul, MN: Redleaf.

Greenman, J. 1998. Parent partnerships: What they don't teach you can hurt. *Child Care Information Exchange* (November/December): 78–82.

Greenspan, S.I., with J. Salmon. 2001. *The four-thirds solution: Solving the child care crisis in America today.* Cambridge, MA: Perseus.

Hahn, T.N. 1996. *The miracle of mindfulness.* Boston: Beacon.

Harms, T., R.M. Clifford, & D. Cryer. 1998a. *Early Childhood Environment Rating Scale.* (ECERS-R). Rev. ed. New York: Teachers College Press.

Harms, T., R.M. Clifford, & D. Cryer. 1998b. *Family Day Care Rating Scale.* New York: Teachers College Press.

Harms, T., R.M. Clifford, & D. Cryer. 1998c. *Infant and Toddler Environment Rating Scale.* New York: Teacher's College Press.

Harms, T., D. Cryer, & R.M. Clifford. 2003. *Infant and Toddler Environment Rating Scale* (ITERS-R). Rev. ed. New York: Teachers College Press.

Head Start Bureau. 1999. *Head Start program performance standards and other regulations.* Washington, DC: U.S. Department of Health and Human Services.

Heffron, M.C. 1999. Balance in jeopardy: Reflexive reactions vs. reflective responses in infant/family practice. *Zero to Three* 20 (1): 15–17.

Hoffman, C. 2000. *The hoop and the tree: A compass for finding deeper relationship with all life.* San Francisco: Council Oak.

Holcomb, B. 1998. *Not guilty! The good news for working mothers.* New York: Touchstone.

Honig, A.S. 2002a. The power of positive attachment. *Scholastic Early Childhood Today* (April): 32–34.

Honig, A.S. 2002b. *Secure relationships: Nurturing infant/toddler attachment in early care settings.* Washington, DC: NAEYC.

Howes, C. 1998. Continuity of care: The importance of infant, toddler, caregiver relationships. *Zero to Three* 18 (6): 7–11.

Howes, C. 1999. Attachment relationships in the context of multiple caregivers. In *Handbook of attachment theory and research,* eds. J. Cassidy & P.R. Shaver, 671–87. New York: Guilford.

Hyun, E. 1998. *Making sense of developmentally and culturally appropriate practice (DCAP) in early childhood education.* New York: Peter Lang.

Jampolsky, G. 1983. *Teach only love.* New York: Bantam.

Josselson, R. 1983. *The space between us: Exploring the dimensions of human relationships.* San Francisco: Jossey-Bass.

Karen, R. 1990. Becoming attached. *Atlantic Monthly* (February): 38.

Karr-Morse, R., & M.S. Wiley. 1997. *Ghosts from the nursery: Tracing the roots of violence.* New York: Atlantic Monthly Press.

Katz, L.G., & D.E. McClellan. 1997. *Fostering children's social competence: The teacher's role.* Washington, DC: NAEYC.

Klaus, M., J.H. Kennell, & P.H. Klaus. 1995. *Bonding: Building the foundations of secure attachments and independence.* New York: Addison-Wesley.

Klein, A.G.S. 2002. Infant and toddler care that recognizes their competence: Practices at the Pikler Institute. *Dimensions of Early Childhood* (Spring): 11–14.

Lally, J.R. 1995, November. The impact of child care policies and practices on infant/toddler identity formation. *Young Children* 51 (1): 58–67.

Lally, J.R. 1998. Brain research, infant learning, and child care curriculum. *Child Care Information Exchange* (May/June): 46–48.

Lally, J.R., A. Griffin, E. Fenichel, M. Segal, E. Szanton, & B. Weissbourd. 1995, 2003. *Caring for infants and toddlers in groups: Developmentally appropriate practice.* Washington, DC: Zero to Three.

Lally, J.R., P. Mangione, & S. Signer. 2002. The importance of intimacy in infant toddler care. Paper presented at the NAEYC Annual Conference, November, New York City.

Lally, J.R., Y.L. Torres, & P.C. Phelps. 1993. *Caring for infants and toddlers in groups: Necessary considerations for emotional, social, and cognitive development.* Washington, DC: Zero to Three. Available online at www.zerotothree.org/caring.html.

Leavitt, R.L. 1994. *Power and emotion in infant toddler care.* Albany, NY: State University Press.

Lee, L., & E. Seiderman. 1998. *The Parent Services Project.* Families Matter series. Cambridge, MA: Harvard Research Project.

Lieberman, A.F. 1993. *The emotional life of the toddler.* New York: Free Press.

Link, G., & M. Beggs, with E. Seiderman. 1997. *Serving families.* Fairfax, CA: Parent Services Project.

Lombardi, J. 2002. *Time to care: Redesigning child care to promote education, support families, and build communities.* Philadelphia, PA: Temple University Press.

Lombardi, J., & J. Poppe. 2001, October. Investing in better care for infants and toddlers: The next frontier for school readiness. NCSL *State Legislative Report* 26 (10). Available online at www.betterbabycare.org/docs/investing.pdf.

Magid, K., & C. McKelvey. 1987. *High risk: Children without a conscience.* New York: Bantam Books.

Malaguzzi, L., & L. Gandini. 1993, November. For an education based on relationships: Reggio Emilia. *Young Children* 49 (1): 9–12.

Mallory, B.L., & R.S. New, eds. 1994. *Diversity and developmentally appropriate practices: Challenges for early childhood education.* New York: Teachers College Press.

Manfredi/Petitt, L.A. 1993, November. Child care: It's more than the sum of its tasks. *Young Children* 49 (1): 40–42.

Manfredi/Petitt, L.A. 2000. Primary caregiving in the early childhood care and education classroom. Handout. Available from the author at Lampetitt@hotmail.com.

Mangione, P.L., ed. 1995. *Infant/toddler caregiving: A guide to culturally sensitive care.* Sacramento, CA: California Department of Education.

Maslow, A. 1970. *Motivation and personality.* New York: Harper and Row.

McCracken, J.B. 1990. So many goodbyes. Brochure. Washington, DC: NAEYC.

Melmed, M. 1997, July. Parents speak: Zero to Three's findings from research on parents' views of early childhood development. Public Policy Report. *Young Children* 52 (5): 46–49.

Miller, K. 1995. Continuity of care: A growing trend. *Child Care Information Exchange* (July/August): 75–76.

Minuchin, P., J. Colapinto, & S. Minuchin. 1998. *Working with families of the poor.* Family Therapy series. New York: Guilford.

Mitchel, A., & J. David, eds. 1992. *Explorations with young children: A curriculum guide from the Bank Street College of Education.* Mt. Ranier, MD: Gryphon House.

Modigliani, K. 1996. *Parents speak about child care: Stressed-out mothers, invisible fathers, and short-changed children.* Families and Work Institute. Boston: Wheelock College.

NAEYC. 1997a, November. *Code of ethical conduct and statement of commitment.* NAEYC Position Statement. Washington, DC: Author. Available online at www.naeyc.org.

NAEYC. 1997b. Developmentally appropriate practice in early childhood programs serving children from birth through age 8. NAEYC Position Statement. In *Developmentally appropriate practice in early childhood programs,* rev. ed., eds. S. Bredekamp and C. Copple, 3–30. Washington, DC: Author. Also available online at www.naeyc.org.

NAEYC. 1998a. *A caring place for your infant.* Brochure, #548. Washington, DC: Author.

NAEYC. 1998b. *Accreditation criteria & procedures of the National Association for the Education of Young Children,* 1998 ed. Washington, DC: Author.

NAEYC. 2004. Final draft: Early childhood program standards and accreditation performance criteria. Available online at www.naeyc.org/accreditation/.

National Association for Family Child Care (NAFCC). 2002. *Quality standards for NAFCC accreditation.* Boston: Author.

National Association of Child Care Resource and Referral Agencies. 1997. Building a partnership with your child care provider. *Daily Parent Newsletter* (Spring): 1–4.

National Institute of Child Health and Human Development (NICHD). 1991. *NICHD study of early child care and youth development.* Rockville, MD: NICHD Information Resource Center. Available online at http://secc.rti.org.

New, R.S. 1999, March. Here, we call it "drop off and pickup": Transition to child care, American style. *Young Children* 54 (2): 34–35.

Ornish, D. 1998. *Love and survival: The scientific basis for the healing power of intimacy.* New York: HarperCollins.

Packard Foundation. 2000. Caring for infants and toddlers. *The Future of Children* 11 (1).

Parent Services Project (PSP). 2001. Parent Services Project and family child care: Extending the community of support. Flyer. Fairfax, CA: Author.

Parent Services Project (PSP). 2001. Working together for children and families. Brochure. San Rafael, CA: Author.

Parlakian, R. 2001. The *power of questions: Building quality relationships with families.* Brochure. Washington, DC: Zero to Three.

Parlakian, R. 2003. *Before the ABCs: Promoting school readiness in infants and toddlers.* Washington, DC: Zero to Three.

Parlakian, R., & N.L. Seibel. 2002. *Building strong foundations.* Washington, DC: Zero to Three.

Pawl, J.H. 1990. Infants in day care: Reflections on experiences, expectations, and relationships. *Zero to Three* 10 (3): 1–6.

Perry, B.D. 1999. Early childhood and brain development. *The Children's Institute International Forum* (Winter): 1–3.

Perry, B.D. 2001. Promoting non-violent behavior in children: The six core strengths. *Scholastic's Early Childhood TODAY* (September): 26–29.

Perry, B.D., L. Hogan, & S.J. Marlin. 2000. Curiosity, pleasure, and play: A neurodevelopmental perspective. *Haaeyc Advocate* (June 15): 1–6.

Piaget, J. 1952. *The origins of intelligence in children.* New York: W.W. Norton.

Piaget, J. 1960. *The child's conception of the world.* Paterson, NJ: Littlefield, Adams.

Pope, J., & E. Seiderman. 2000–01. The child care connection. *America's Family Support Magazine* (Winter): 23–35.

Porter, L.L. 2003. The science of attachment, the biological roots of love. *Mothering* (July/August): 60–70.

Program for Infant/Toddler Caregivers (PITC). 1996. Booklet accompanying *Protective urges* video. Sacramento, CA: WestEd.

Program for Infant/Toddler Caregivers (PITC). 1997. *PITC trainers manual, Module IV: Culture, family, and providers.* Rev. ed. Sacramento, CA: WestEd.

Pulaski, M.A.S. 1980. *Understanding Piaget.* New York: Harper & Row.

Raikes, H. 1993. Relationship duration in infant care: Time with a high ability teacher and infant-teacher attachment. *Early Childhood Research Quarterly* 8: 309–25.

Raikes, H. 1996, July. A secure base for babies: Applying attachment concepts to the infant care setting. *Young Children* 51 (5): 59–67.

Ready for School Goal Team. 2000. School readiness in North Carolina. Greensboro, NC: SERVE & University of North Carolina. Available online at www.serve.org/publications/NCFull%20Report.pdf.

Regional Educational Laboratories' Early Childhood Collaboration Network. 1995. *Continuity in early childhood: A framework for home, school, and community linkages.*

Oak Brook, IL: North Central Regional Educational Laboratory. Available online at www.sedl.org/prep/hsclinkages.pdf.

Rodriguez, G.G. 1999. *Raising nuestros ninos: Bringing up Latino children in a bicultural world.* New York: Fireside.

Rogers, F. 1998. Keynote address. NAEYC Annual Conference, November 18, Toronto, Canada.

Satir, V. 1972. *Peoplemaking: Because you want to be a better parent.* Palo Alto, CA: Science and Behavior Books.

Satir, V. 1976. *Making contact.* Berkeley, CA: Celestial Arts.

Seibel, N.L. 2003. How to develop the minds, hearts, and capacities of those who work with families. *America's Family Support Magazine* (Spring/Summer): 38–39.

Selection Research Inc. (SRI). 1989. *The Early Childhood Teacher Perceiver.* Lincoln, NE: Author.

SERVE Regional Educational Laboratory. 2001. *Building babies' brains: A training for infant/toddler caregivers.* Trainer's guide. Greensboro, NC: SERVE and University of North Carolina. Available online at www.serve.org/publications/ecbbt.pdf.

Shore, R. 1997. *Rethinking the brain: New insights into early development.* New York: Families and Work Institute.

Small, M.F. 1998. *Our babies, ourselves. How biology and culture shape the way we parent.* New York: Anchor.

Stewart, P. 2000a. *Leave a legacy.* South Hamilton, MA: Compassion Company.

Stewart, P. 2000b. *Living with love.* South Hamilton, MA: Compassion Company.

Stoddard, A. 1997. *Living in love.* New York: William Morrow.

Streeter, B.U., & T.F. Barrett. 1999. *Consultation with day care centers: Supporting quality care for preschool aged children.* Cleveland, OH: Cleveland Center for Research in Child Development.

Swick, K.J. 1991. Teacher-parent partnerships to enhance school success in early childhood education. Washington, DC: National Education Association. *ERIC Digest* ED351149. Available online at www.ericfacility.net/ericdigests/ed351149.html.

Sylwester, R. 1995. A celebration of neurons: An educator's guide to the human brain. Alexandria, VA: Association for Supervision and Curriculum Development.

Tannen, D. 1990. *You just don't understand: Women and men in conversation.* New York: Ballantine.

Unell, B.C., & J.L. Wyckoff. 2000. *The eight seasons of parenthood. How the stages of parenting constantly reshape our adult identities.* New York: Time Books.

Van IJzendoorn, M.H., A. Sagi, & M. Lambermon. 1992. The multiple caregiver paradox: Data from Holland and Israel. In *Beyond the parent: The role of other adults in children's lives,* ed. R.C. Pianta, 5-27. New Directions for Child Development, no. 57. San Francisco: Jossey-Bass.

Whitebook, M., C. Howes, & D. Phillips. 1990. *Who cares? Child care teachers and the quality of care in America. Executive summary, National Child Care Staffing Study.* Washington, DC: Child Care Employee Project (now the Center for the Child Care Workforce).

Whitehead, L.C., & S.I. Ginsberg. 1999, March. Creating a family-like atmosphere in child care settings: All the more difficult in large child care centers. *Young Children* 54 (2): 4–10.

Whitehead, S. 2002. Child care today: What kids need and why so few get it. *Atlanta Our Kids* (February): 19–22.

Winnicott, D.W. 1986. *Home is where we start from: Essays by a psychoanalyst.* New York: W.W. Norton.

Winnicott, D.W. 1987. *Babies and their mothers.* Reading, MA: Addison-Wesley.

Wright, K. 1997, October. Babies, bonds, and brains. *Discover* 18 (10): 75–77.

Zero to Three. 1992. *Heart Start: The emotional foundations of school readiness.* Washington, DC: Author.

Organizations and websites

Better Brains for Babies. ph 706-542-7566 (Diane Bales, project director). www.bbbgeorgia.org

Children's Foundation, Washington, DC. ph: 202-347-3300. www.childrensfoundation.net

Family Support America, Chicago, IL. ph 312-338-0900. www.familysupportamerica.org

Head Start Information and Publication Center (HSIPC), Washington, DC. ph 866-763-6481. www.headstartinfo.org

National Association for the Education of Young Children (NAEYC), Washington, DC. toll free 1-800-424-2460. www.naeyc.org

National Association for Family Child Care (NAFCC), Salt Lake City, UT. toll free 1-801-262-3295. www.nafcc.org

National Resource Center for Health and Safety in Child Care (NRCHSCC), Denver, CO. toll free 1-800-598-5437. http://nrc.uchsc.edu/

Parent Services Project (PSP), San Rafael, CA. ph 415-454-1870. www.parentservices.org

Program for Infant/Toddler Caregivers (PITC), a collaboration of the California Board of Education and WestEd, Sausalito, CA. ph 415-289-2300. www.pitc.org

RC[3] (Relationship-Centered Child Care), Child Care Group, Dallas, TX. toll free 1-888-824-4538. www.childcaregroup.org

WestEd, Center for Child and Family Studies, San Francisco, CA. toll free 1-877-493-7833. www.wested.org

Zero to Three: National Center for Infants, Toddlers, and Families, Washington, DC. ph 202-638-1144. www.zerotothree.org

> Better Baby Care: A Partnership Project of Zero to Three. www.betterbabycare.org

> Early Head Start National Resource Center @ Zero to Three. www.ehsnrc.org

Early years are learning years

Become a member of NAEYC, and help make them count!

Just as you help young children learn and grow, the National Association for the Education of Young Children—your professional organization—supports you in the work you love. NAEYC is the world's largest early childhood education organization, with a national network of local, state, and regional Affiliates. We are more than 100,000 members working together to bring high-quality early learning opportunities to all children from birth through age 8.

Since 1926, NAEYC has provided educational services and resources for people working with children, including:

• *Young Children*, the award-winning journal (six issues a year) for early childhood educators

• **Books, posters, brochures, and videos** to support your work with young children and families

• **The NAEYC Annual Conference**, which brings tens of thousands of people together from across the country and around the world to share their expertise and ideas on the education of young children

• **Insurance plans** for members and programs

• **A voluntary accreditation system** to help programs reach national standards for high-quality early childhood education

• **Young Children International** to promote global communication and information exchanges

• **www.naeyc.org**—a dynamic Web site with up-to-date information on all of our services and resources

To join NAEYC

To find a complete list of membership benefits and options or to join NAEYC online, visit **www.naeyc.org/membership.** Or you can mail this form to us.

(Membership must be for an individual, not a center or school.)

Name _____

Address _____

City_____ State_____ ZIP_____

E-mail _____

Phone (H)_____ (W)_____

❏ New member

❏ Renewal ID # _____

Affiliate name/number _____

To determine your dues, you must visit **www.naeyc.org/membership** or call 800-424-2460, ext. 2002.

Indicate your payment option

❏ VISA ❏ MasterCard ❏ AmEx ❏ Discover

Card # _____

Exp. date _____

Cardholder's name _____

Signature _____

Note: By joining NAEYC you can also become a member of your state and local Affiliates.

Send this form and payment to

NAEYC
PO Box 97156
Washington, DC 20090-7156